PSORIASIS &
ECZEMA

PSORIASIS & ECZEMA

EDITED BY LIONEL FRY

CONSULTANT DERMATOLOGIST
ST. MARY'S HOSPITAL
LONDON

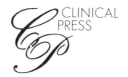

CLINICAL
PRESS

Published by Clinical Press Limited. Registered Office: The Coach House, 26 Oakfield Road, Clifton, Bristol BS8 2AT

British Library Cataloguing in Publication Data

Psoriasis and eczema.
  1. Eczema   2. Psoriasis
  I. Fry, L.
  616.5′21   RL251

  ISBN 1–85457–002–1

Library of Congress Cataloging-in-Publication Data

Psoriasis and eczema / edited by L. Fry.
     p.   cm.
  Includes bibliographies and index.
  ISBN 1–85457–002–1: £20.00 (U.K.: est.)
  1. Psoriasis. 2. Eczema. I. Fry, Lionel.
  [DNLM: 1. Eczema. 2. Psoriasis. WR 205 P9715]
  RL321.P738 1988
  616.5′21—dc 19
  DNLM/DLC
  for Library of Congress   87—32500
                            CIP

Typeset, printed and bound in Great Britain by Butler & Tanner Ltd, Frome and London

Contents

Preface   vi

1 Psoriasis: Clinical Features
   L. Fry   1

2 The Treatment of Psoriasis
   C. E. M. Griffiths   39

3 The Aetiology and Pathogenesis of Psoriasis
   B. S. Baker   65

4 Eczema: Clinical Features
   R. J. Clayton   105

5 The Management of Eczema
   J. N. Leonard   123

6 The Aetiology of Eczema
   A. V. Powles   161

   Index   195

Preface

Both psoriasis and eczema are common skin disorders and constitute a large proportion of consultations in both general practice and a dermatology clinic in hospital practice. The cause of these disorders has so far eluded the investigators, although the treatments have improved over the last two decades. However these improvements have been largely empirical rather than based on scientific deduction. Fortunately our understanding of the biological abnormalities in eczema and psoriasis has increased as a result of the development of new scientific techniques. It is a personal opinion, but I feel that greater advances have been made in our knowledge of psoriasis than in the constitutional eczemas. This book, therefore, is intended to give some insight into recent advances in the pathogenicity of these diseases as well as their clinical features and management.

It is a pleasure to acknowledge my co-authors in this text, all of whom are from the Dermatology Unit at St Mary's, and particularly Dr D S Baker, who is a scientist and not a clinician, and who, in collaboration with Professor Helgi Valdimarsson, has made a significant contribution to our understanding of psoriasis.

LIONEL FRY

1

PSORIASIS: CLINICAL FEATURES

L. Fry

The term psoriasis comes from the Greek word meaning to itch, and was first used by Galen, who described a scaly itchy rash on the eyelids and genitalia, which was probably not psoriasis as we know it today, but eczema. Description of a skin disorder compatible with psoriasis is present in the Old Testament. Interestingly, it appears that psoriasis was grouped with leprosy by the Greeks and subsequently, until the nineteenth century. This grouping led to psoriatics being rejected by the community, and there are reports of their being burned at the stake in the fourteenth century. It was not until the first half of the nineteenth century that psoriasis was described as a separate and definite clinical entity.

EPIDEMIOLOGY

Incidence

Data relating to the incidence of psoriasis worldwide are not precise. The disease appears to be most common in northern European countries and amongst Europeans of the USA. It

1

has been shown to be rare amongst the American Indians, uncommon in mongoloid Asians and Negroes of West Africa, but there is a higher incidence in the Negroes of East Africa. Recent reports on Arabs have given an incidence similar to that of northern European countries, the Hindus in the subcontinent of India have an incidence approaching 1% which is less than Europeans, but higher than Asians from the Far East.

In the UK approximately 2% of the population have psoriasis. In a classical study in the Faroe Islands when one-third of the population were seen, the incidence was found to be 2.84%[1].

Social Groups

Psoriasis appears to have a similar incidence in all social groups in the UK.

Sex Incidence

Although there are some reports which have shown a higher incidence in one sex, it is generally agreed that the sex incidence is similar for psoriasis.

GENETICS

Family Studies

There is no doubt that genetic factors are important in the aetiology of psoriasis. It has been found in large surveys[2] that one-third of patients have a positive family history. A heritable process in 80% of psoriatic families over a 75-year period was demonstrated in the town of Wurzberg[3]. Psoriasis is three times more common in psoriatic siblings one of whose parents has the disease, than when neither parent is affected.

Studies on twins support strong inheritance factors in psoriasis. The most important study was carried out in Denmark, in which 36 pairs were seen, one of whom at least had psoriasis[4]. There were 14 monozygotic and 22 dizygotic like-sexed pairs. The pair-wise concordance rate, which gives the number of pairs in which both partners have psoriasis out of the total number in the group, is 0.64 in the monozygotic and 0.14 in the dizygotic group. The proband-wise concordance rate (risk of psoriasis in partners of twin patients with the disease) was 0.72 in monozygotic and 0.17 in dizygotic pairs. The study also showed that the clinical type of psoriasis, age of onset, course and severity of the disease is influenced by genetic factors.

HLA Studies

The class I antigens B13, B17, B37[5] and Cw6[6] are significantly increased in psoriasis. A positive association with B16 has been found in France and the USA but not in the Scandinavian countries. B13, B17 and B37 are in linkage disequilibrium with Cw6, and may well account for the grouping in psoriasis. More recently the class II antigen DR7 has been shown to be increased in psoriasis, and it has been suggested that both Cw6 and DR7 are the genes associated with the disease.

Certainly not all patients with psoriasis have the same HLA phenotype, and it is likely that a number of different genes are responsible for the clinical expression of the disease. B13, B17 and B37 have been found to be associated with early onset of the disease, and with guttate psoriasis. The latter is the pattern of psoriasis triggered by streptococcal infections, and it has been shown that patients who have B13 are more likely to have an exacerbation after streptococcal infections. So called pustular psoriasis of the palms and soles is a distinct clinical entity (see below) and its relationship to plaque psoriasis is still debatable. An increase of AW19 and BW35 have been found in pustular psoriasis[7] but not B13, B17 and B37. This would imply that psoriasis and pustular psoriasis may be different diseases, and the term pustular psoriasis is therefore misleading.

Psoriatic arthropathy has an increased incidence of B27, as has Reiter's disease and ankylosing spondylitis, and there may well be a strong pathogenic link between these disorders.

However, as with other disorders with significantly increased incidences of certain histocompatibility antigens, the association in psoriasis and its clinical variations is not 100%. This probably implies that these particular histocompatibility genes are not the ones responsible for the pathological changes, but are closely related to the actual disease genes on the chromosomes. The HLA and family studies at present imply multifactorial inheritance due to several genes. A small number of genes may be the important ones determining the predisposition to the disease, but there are in addition likely to be a number of modifying genes which determine whether psoriasis appears and what clinical form it may take. However, the so-called 'principal' or determining genes which predispose to the disease do appear to be inherited as dominant rather than recessive ones.

MORPHOLOGY OF THE LESION

The typical psoriatic lesion is a raised red scaly patch with a sharply demarcated edge, between the clinically uninvolved skin and the plaque (Figures 1.1 and 1.2). The size of these lesions varies from a few millimetres to several centimetres, and there may be large confluent areas of psoriasis on the trunk or limbs. On rare occasions this may extend to involve all the skin (erythrodermic psoriasis – see below).

If the scale is thick the plaque has a greyish-white colour. However, if the scale is not too thick the patch of psoriasis has a predominantly red colour. If the plaque is excoriated with a wooden spatula (grattage) the red patch develops a white flaky surface as the scale in psoriasis is loosely bound. This is a useful sign in distinguishing psoriasis from other dermatoses. Another useful sign is removal of all the scale by more vigorous excoriation with the spatula, then a red glistening surface with capillary bleeding points appears. Occasionally, when the scaling and plaque is very thick, deep fissures develop, which can be painful.

A rare form of psoriasis are the so-called rupioid lesions. These are thicker than common plaque psoriasis and have a conical shape. They have a yellowish-brown colour and are most frequently seen on the feet; the appearance is produced by a thicker and more adherent scale, which becomes heaped.

CLINICAL PATTERNS

Although there are various clinical patterns psoriasis tends to be a symmetrical eruption (Figures 1.1–1.3). Unilateral lesions do occur, but if this is the presentation it is important to carefully consider other conditions which are more likely to be asymmetrical.

Plaque Psoriasis

This is the commonest form of psoriasis. Characteristically the plaques occur on the extensor surfaces of the knees and elbows (Figure 1.1). The lesions tend to be discoid or coin shaped (Figures 1.1 and 1.3). The size may vary from one to several centimetres in diameter. Other common sites to be involved are the scalp, particularly behind the ears, and the sacral region. The extent of plaque psoriasis may vary from the single lesion on each elbow or knee, to numerous plaques all over the body. The face is an uncommon site to be involved.

Guttate Psoriasis

Guttate comes from the Latin word 'gutta' meaning 'a drop'. In guttate psoriasis the lesions appear suddenly usually over the upper trunk, (Figure 1.4), although the limbs, face and scalp may be affected. The lesions are smaller than in plaque psoriasis and tend to vary from 1 to 10 mm. However, the lesions have the same characteristics as those in the plaque disease.

Guttate psoriasis is most commonly seen in children and young adults and typically follows a streptococcal upper respiratory tract infection. The psoriasis lesions appear 2–3 weeks after the streptococcal infection and new lesions may continue to appear for up to a month from the onset of the eruption. Spontaneous resolution usually occurs after 2–3 months. Occasionally guttate psoriasis may transform to plaque disease.

Guttate psoriasis often occurs in patients with no pre-existing lesions, but it does also occur in patients with existing plaque disease. In the latter instance the guttate lesions may clear after 3 months, but the plaques may remain.

Erythrodermic Psoriasis

Erythrodermic is the term used to denote 100% involvement of the skin surface (Figure 1.5). It may occur in diseases other than psoriasis, notably eczema and skin lymphomas. In erythrodermic psoriasis the skin is redder (as the name implies) and the thick white scaling is usually not present. The scales appear to be shed more rapidly instead of being heaped up and retained, although the surface of the skin is scaly.

Erythrodermic psoriasis is usually preceded by chronic plaque disease, which gradually becomes more extensive and finally erythrodermic. However, the time from progression of the plaque to erythrodermic disease is variable, and has been found to be from 1 month to 34 years. The incidence of

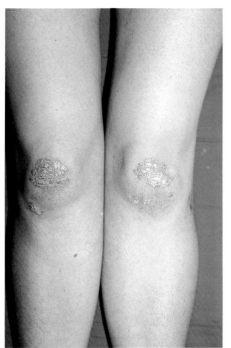

Figure 1.1 Symmetrical well-demarcated plaques of psoriasis on the knees

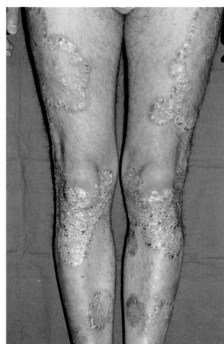

Figure 1.2 Extensive plaques of psoriasis on the legs

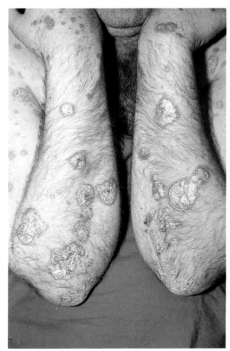

Figure 1.3 Symmetrical plaques of psoriasis on the arms

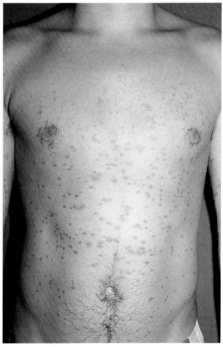

Figure 1.4 Guttate psoriasis

facing p. 6

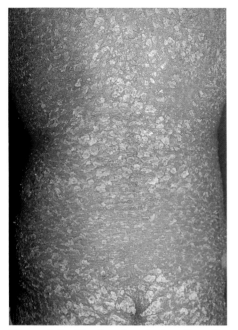

Figure 1.5 Erythrodermic (confluent) psoriasis

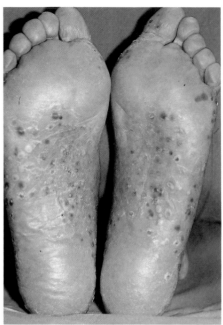

Figure 1.6 Localized pustular psoriasis on the soles

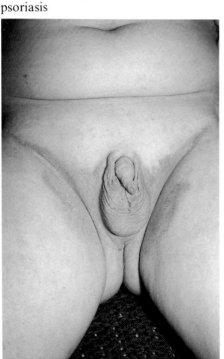

Figure 1.7 Intertriginous or flexural psoriasis in a child; this is a common site for psoriasis in children

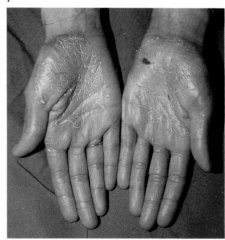

Figure 1.8 Confluent symmetrical involvement on the palms

erythrodermic psoriasis is less than 1% of all forms of the disease, and is usually in young and middle-aged adults.

Pustular Psoriasis

As the name implies this form of psoriasis is associated with pustules as part of the morphology. There are two distinct forms of pustular psoriasis.

Generalized pustular psoriasis The onset is acute with areas of erythema which are scaly at the edge, and sheets of small pustules developing in the erythematous areas. The eruption is widespread and associated with constitutional upset, the patient feeling ill and having a raised temperature. The disease usually subsides after a few weeks, but patients are liable to further episodes. Pustular psoriasis usually occurs in those with established plaque or occasionally guttate psoriasis. In a small proportion, approximately 15%, generalized pustular psoriasis is preceded by localized pustular psoriasis on the palms and soles, or on the tips of the digits.

A number of precipitating factors have been incriminated for converting stable plaque disease into generalized pustular psoriasis, and these are discussed below. It may well be that there are genetic factors predisposing to pustular psoriasis. This type of eruption may be seen at any age, but its highest incidence is the middle-aged and the elderly.

Localized pustular psoriasis As mentioned above, it is debatable whether localized pustular psoriasis is part of the psoriasis spectrum or a separate entity. The term localized pustular psoriasis is reserved for a characteristic eruption which occurs on the palms and soles; it is sometimes referred to as palmoplantar pustulosis. The features are of well-demarcated red scaling areas with small pustules (Figure 1.6). The pustules are sterile. The disorder may be symmetrical or unilateral, and may affect only the palms or soles or both.

Localized pustular psoriasis is very persistent; one survey found only 28% of patients clear and in remission after a 10-

year follow-up[8]. It is more common in females, the M/F ratio being 1:3. It most frequently begins in young and middle-aged adults; approximately 10% of patients have features of classical plaque psoriasis elsewhere.

Acrodermatitis continua This rather cumbersome term applies to a form of pustular psoriasis which begins on the tips of the fingers or toes. Initially there is erythema around the nails, minimal scaling ensues and there is frequently swelling of the nail fold, mimicking chronic paronychia. Small pustules then appear around the nails and in the nail bed. The condition usually starts on one digit and gradually spreads to involve others. There is frequently destruction of the nail plate once the disease becomes established.

Acrodermatitis continua usually begins either in children or in the elderly. In children it may go into remission after some years, whereas in the elderly it is persistent and may eventually spread and evolve into plaque or generalized psoriasis.

Acrodermatitis continua is a very rare form of psoriasis, the incidence being less than 0.5% of patients with all forms of the disease.

MORPHOLOGY AT SPECIFIC SITES

Scalp

Psoriasis may be localized to the scalp with no involvement elsewhere. There may be discrete plaques or there may be confluent patches covering large areas of the scalp, or the whole of the scalp may be affected. There is usually a sharp cut-off at the hair-line, between involvement of the scalp and the non-hair-bearing skin. This is a characteristic feature.

The scales of the psoriatic patches in scalp involvement may become attached to the hairs and heaped up, forming exceptionally thick scaly plaques. Hair loss is rare in scalp involvement, but has been described, and usually takes the form of thinning of the hair rather than complete hair loss in an affected area.

Flexural or Intertriginous Psoriasis

Psoriasis may occur solely at intertriginous sites, or at these sites with plaque psoriasis elsewhere. Intertriginous psoriasis involving the perianal skin and genitalia is a common presentation in children. In adults perianal skin involvement may be the sole feature of the disease.

Because of the moisture in the intertriginous areas the dry flaky appearance is lost and the psoriasis presents as a firm red smooth plaque with a shiny surface. Once again the sharp line of demarcation between the plaque and uninvolved skin should suggest the diagnosis (Figure 1.7). Another common feature of intertrigenous psoriasis is deep painful fissures that may occur at the apex of the skin folds.

Differential Diagnosis
(Intertriginous psoriasis)

● Seborrhoeic eczema
● Erythrasma
● Fungal infections

Palms and Soles

Psoriasis presenting at these sites often has a different appearance from psoriasis elsewhere on the body. Apart from the rupioid lesions mentioned above, the involvement may be as thickening and redness without the typical white thick scale, but only a fine scale. The disease on the palms and soles is often as a confluent area of the whole palm or sole, with once again a sharp line of demarcation between involved and non-involved skin (Figure 1.8). Painful fissures are often present in the skin creases. The thickening of the skin may lead to loss of mobility and severe impairment of function of the hand.

Mucosal Lesions

Oral lesions are extremely rare. When present the lesions are small yellowish-white plaques on the tongue, palate and buccal mucosa.

Ocular lesions that may occur, but usually only in widespread and erythrodermic psoriasis, include blepharitis and keratitis.

Penile lesions occur in both circumcised and uncircumcised individuals. The glans penis is the most common site and the lesions consist of small red plaques, scaly in the circumcised and with a shiny surface in the uncircumcised.

NAILS

Nail involvement is fairly common in psoriasis, with approximately one-third of all patients showing some nail changes. As a general rule nail changes are seen more frequently in patients with extensive disease or in patients with psoriatic arthropathy. Finger nails are more frequently affected than toe nails. The type of nail abnormality seen depends on whether the psoriatic process has affected the nail matrix or nail bed.

Pitting

This is the commonest nail abnormality with resulting malformation of the plate. It is due to psoriatic involvement of the nail matrix. The pits are small pin-sized lesions (Figure 1.9).

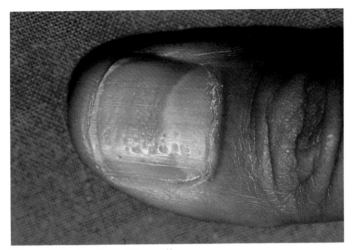

Figure 1.9 Pitting of the nail

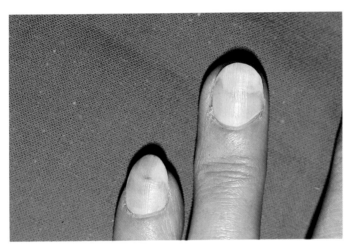

Figure 1.10 Onycholysis

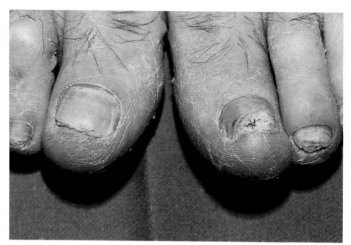

Figure 1.11 Severe nail dystrophy in psoriasis with gross subungual hyperkeratosis

Onycholysis

This is lifting of the nail plate from the nail bed when there is involvement of the latter. Clinically this presents as lifting of the terminal part of the plate with extension of the white opaque colour proximally (Figure 1.10). The onycholysis may be extensive with lifting of the whole plate and its subsequent loss. However, if this does occur a new nail plate will form, but there will almost certainly be onycholysis again. Only one, or all, the fingernails may be affected.

Discolorations

Brownish-red discolorations of the nail bed with an 'oil drop' appearance are due to small patches of psoriasis on the nail bed. Splinter haemorrhages may also occur due to increased capillary fragility of the enlarged capillaries in the psoriatic process.

Nail Dystrophy

If the involvement of the nail matrix is severe then a whitish crumbly nail plate is produced.

Subungual Hyperkeratosis

This is heaping-up of the abnormal keratin from the nail bed when there is severe and extensive involvement of the nail bed (Figure 1.11).

AGE OF ONSET

Psoriasis may begin at any age. However, it is rare before the age of 5. The average age of onset has been found to be in the 20s in most large studies; 10% of patients have an onset before 10, 35% before 20, and 58% before 30. However, the average age of onset is not the same in the different clinical patterns of psoriasis. This may be due to different genetic and/or environmental factors which determine the clinical expression of the disease, and age of onset is one of them.

SYMPTOMS

In the majority of patients psoriasis gives rise to very few physical symptoms. It is likely to lead to many more psycho-social problems (see below) because of appearance of the rash.

Itch

A small proportion of patients, approximately 5–10%, will complain of irritation. Only in a minority of these does the irritation become severe enough to warrant specific anti-itch therapy. If the itch is severe then active treatment to clear psoriasis is the best approach.

Pain

Psoriasis will cause pain if the skin splits and fissures develop. Fissures are most commonly seen in flexural and intertriginous psoriasis, thick plaque psoriasis over joints, and in severe psoriasis on the palms and soles.

Scaling

Patients often complain bitterly of the excessive scaling of the skin. When there is scalp involvement this gives rise to 'dandruff' on the clothes. When there is extensive involvement of the skin, patients produce a shower of scale when they take their clothes off, and they will find it too embarrassing to go to hotels or stay with friends. Some get over this problem by taking a small vacuum cleaner or dustpan and brush with them.

Loss of Mobility

Confluent psoriasis over joints may lead to lack of mobility, as psoriasis is not as pliable as normal skin. This may be a severe problem when the hands are involved.

Shivering

This occurs in erythrodermic psoriasis. Patients lose a great deal of heat in this form of the disease because of the increased blood flow through the skin.

Constitutional Upset

Fever and malaise occur with generalized pustular psoriasis.

Psychosocial Aspect

In the majority of patients the appearance of the rash is the only 'side-effect'. What effect the rash has on the patient usually depends on the personality of the individual. Many patients with severe disease appear to cope well, whilst others with minimal involvement find it difficult to accept the disability. Obviously if the rash is visible, i.e. on the hands or face, then this may well lead to greater problems.

In the majority of patients with psoriasis there will be some withdrawal from social contacts. Apart from the appearance there is a still widely held belief by the non-sufferers that psoriasis is a contagious disorder, and therefore sufferers should be avoided. This, in addition to the appearance of the rash, leads to isolation. The age of onset of psoriasis is important in the degree of harm it may cause socially. The adolescent will have more problems adjusting than the mature adult in a family situation. Psoriasis has also been shown, not surprisingly, to have an effect on sexual behaviour, the effect being greater upon women. The majority of patients will not indulge in sporting activity, particularly swimming, and many, for this reason, will not take holidays in the sun and sea.

Psoriasis may also lead to problems with employment if there is involvement of the hands and face. Occupations involving coming into contact with the public will be difficult in this situation.

The two psychological disorders which are increased in psoriasis are depression and obsessional states. These would appear to be the direct result of the physical disability in the subject with a possible predisposition to these states.

NATURAL HISTORY AND PROGNOSIS

Psoriasis runs a variable course, and it is not possible to predict if and when spontaneous resolution may occur, if the disease will remain static, or whether it will become more extensive. However, the various clinical patterns of psoriasis tend to have different prognoses. Plaque psoriasis, which begins in childhood and adolescence, tends to have a poorer prognosis than late-onset disease, and it is more likely to be persistent. Other poor prognostic signs are extent of disease and appearance of new lesions. When the rash is very widespread remissions are less likely to ensue. If the patient finds the involvement is gradually increasing then remission is unlikely in the near future.

In long-term follow-up studies of patients with plaque psoriasis[9], the incidence of spontaneous remission has been found to be approximately 40%. The length of remissions after treatment depends on a number of inherent variable factors in the psoriatic process (see below – disease activity), and are not necessarily dependent on nature of the treatment. It has often been reported that the lesions reappear more rapidly after topical treatment with steroids compared to dithranol, but this is a generalization which certainly is not true in all individuals. In very active disease the lesions will reappear within 2–3 weeks of stopping treatment, whatever modality is employed. At present no particular treatment is more likely to give longer remission than others currently available. The speed, extent and incidence of relapse depends on disease activity and not the treatment. In addition it is not possible to predict which treatment will prove the most effective in clearing the lesions.

Guttate psoriasis usually has a good prognosis, and in over 95% of patients the eruption will disappear within 3–4 months of onset. Occasionally guttate psoriasis may convert into plaque disease and the prognosis is then that of the latter, which is unpredictable and variable. Patients who have had one attack of guttate psoriasis are likely to develop further episodes if they have infections with the streptococcus or certain viruses. Prophylactic penicillin should be considered if the attacks are frequent, and can be shown to have been due to streptococcal infections.

Guttate psoriasis may occur in individuals who have no previous lesions, or those who have plaque disease. In the latter the guttate lesions clear after 3–4 months, but the plaque disease invariably persists.

The prognosis in erythrodermic psoriasis tends to be poor. Patients with this form of the disease need active treatment often with systemic drugs. The natural history is therefore modified by treatment. The majority of patients after the active phase may revert to extensive chronic plaque disease, which again usually requires long-term active systemic therapy or psoralens and ultraviolet A (PUVA) therapy. Erythrodermic phases are likely to recur, unless there is an identifiable course which can be prevented, or patients are maintained on indefinite systemic therapy.

Generalized pustular psoriasis has a risk of death. In one series[10] of 106 patients there were 26 deaths attributable to the disease or its therapy. The acute episode of pustulation may last many weeks, but it is now modified with therapy. Once the pustular phase has subsided the condition usually reverts to the chronic plaque state. However, further bouts of acute pustular psoriasis associated with acrodermatitis continua tend to have a bad prognosis.

Localized pustular psoriasis on the palms and soles tends to be very persistent. Over a 10-year period only approximately 25% of patients are likely to achieve a remission. The disease, however, is not commonly seen in the elderly, so presumably spontaneous remission does occur but only after some 20–30 years.

Acrodermatitis continua (pustular involvement around the nails and on the nail bed) has a poor prognosis in the elderly. The condition is very persistent and not responsive to treatment, and usually gradually progresses to widespread plaque disease, with a tendency to generalized pustular psoriasis.

Nail abnormalities often run a similar course to the skin lesions. If the skin disease is persistent then the nail problems are also likely to persist. Occasionally nail involvement is seen without skin lesions, and this again has a variable prognosis. The lesions may persist for years, or there may be spontaneous remission with subsequent relapse. Unfortunately nail abnormalities do not respond to topical remedies, and thus systemic drugs, PUVA, or intra-lesional steroids to nail beds are required, and these are not without morbidity.

In considering the prognosis of the disease it is necessary to take into account not only the natural history, but also the morbidity and even fatalities caused by the currently available therapies. As the drugs and other modalities become more

effective they often bring added risks, and drugs used in psoriasis are no exception. Potent topical steroids may cause a
number of cutaneous problems if used incorrectly, and
dithranol may cause some burning and blister formation.
Long-term PUVA causes changes in the skin, and the risk of
cutaneous malignancies is still to be assessed. The systemic
drugs (retinoids, methotrexate and cyclosporin) currently
employed all have serious potential side-effects, particularly if
used long-term, and thus there is increased morbidity and even
fatality from treatment. These problems have to be taken into
account when considering the prognosis.

PRECIPITATING FACTORS

There are a number of known precipitating factors in psoriasis.
However, not all will precipitate or exacerbate the disease in
different individuals. It appears that there are modifying
factors in different patients which govern whether lesions will
be produced in a given instance.

Precipitating Factors

- Infections
- Hormonal
- Psychogenic
- Drugs
- Physical trauma

Infections

Streptococcal infection is probably the most definite known
trigger. The pattern of disease produced by streptococcal infections is guttate psoriasis. Patients with established chronic
plaque psoriasis may develop an acute flare-up which is similar

to the guttate-type eruption on the trunk and limbs. It has recently been shown that monoclonal antibodies derived from streptococcal antigens will bind to epitopes on the keratinocytes. This would explain how the streptococcus could initiate pathology in susceptible individuals. Other upper respiratory tract infections, probably viral, also appear to be able to cause guttate psoriasis. There is no strong association between other known infections and psoriasis.

Hormonal factors

Female sex hormones appear to be able to influence psoriasis. An increased incidence of onset has been reported at both puberty and the menopause. Pregnancy usually has a beneficial effect (50% of patients in one series reported improvement during pregnancy). Hypoparathyroidism (and other causes of a low serum calcium) have been shown to exacerbate psoriasis. There is a strong link between many endogenous hormones and the immune system, and it is likely that the changes in the hormones, be they physiological or pathological, influence psoriasis by their effect on immunological pathways in the skin.

Psychogenic Factors

There is no doubt that in a proportion of patients psychogenic stress does appear to precipitate or exacerbate psoriasis. However, there are reports which did not find any convincing evidence that stress plays a part in the cause or persistence of psoriasis. It is difficult to measure stress and how different individuals react to it. It is well established that stress does influence the endocrine system, which in turn effects immunological responses, as occur in psoriasis. It would appear that, like other triggers, stress may be an aggravating factor in some but not all patients. It is likely that the modifying factors (which are probably genetically determined) and which may influence the response to specific triggers, such as stress, are not uniform in the psoriatic population.

Drugs

Lithium   Lithium is now an established drug in psychiatry and may aggravate plaque and localized pustular psoriasis. It is probably now the most common drug to exacerbate psoriasis. It appears lithium exacerbates existing disease rather than precipitates it.

Antimalarials   Chloroquine and mepacrine have both been reported to exacerbate psoriasis, but considering their widespread use in the past, they appear rarely to affect psoriasis.

Non-steroidal anti-inflammatory drugs   Indomethacin has been reported to exacerbate existing disease, although it is widely used by rheumatologists for psoriatic arthropathy. Certainly indomethacin and other non-steroidal anti-inflammatory drugs do not aggravate the disease in every psoriatic patient who takes them.

β-blockers   In a small proportion of patients these drugs do appear to worsen psoriasis. However, because the incidence of this side-effect is so low, psoriasis should not be considered as a contraindication to their use.

Systemic corticosteroids   This group of drugs has a beneficial effect on psoriasis, but when the dose is reduced, or the drug stopped, there may be a rebound exacerbation of the disease. For this reason systemic steroids should not be used in the treatment of psoriasis. Very severe exacerbations, including erythroderma and generalized pustular psoriasis, have been reported after their use.

Trauma

It has been known for over 100 years that localized trauma to the skin may precipitate psoriasis in a proportion of patients. This was described by Heinrich Koebner in 1878 and since that time it has been known as the *Koebner phenomenon*. The psoriasis appears some 2–4 weeks after trauma to the skin, precisely at the site of the injury. The nature of the injury is not important providing there is damage to the epidermis. The Koebner phenomenon is seen after cuts, grazes and burns. It may also be seen after damage to the skin from other skin diseases, such as herpes zoster, impetigo, fungal infections and eczema. Sunlight, which usually has a beneficial effect on psoriasis, will also induce psoriasis if the patient damages the skin by 'sunburn'.

Only a minority of patients are so-called Koebner-positive, i.e. injury to the skin induces psoriasis. The incidence of Koebner-positive patients is approximately 25% of all psoriatics, and it is an 'all-or-none' phenomenon, i.e. damage to the skin at any site will induce psoriasis, whilst in the Koebner-negative patient injury at any site has no effect. These observations would seem to imply a humoral factor, which is responsible for the positive or negative outcome to trauma.

Epidemiological studies on the Koebner phenomenon have looked at whether a particular type of psoriasis is more likely to be associated with a positive response. The results are conflicting but guttate psoriasis does appear to have a higher incidence of positivity. It has also been found that patients whose psoriasis begins at an early age are more likely to be positive.

The Koebner phenomenon is probably more important for research than as a clinical entity. The Koebner response is a model in which the evolution of psoriasis may be studied, and may well tell us a great deal about the disease.

DISEASE ACTIVITY

The word 'active' is often used to describe psoriasis, when new lesions are appearing and the disease becoming more extensive. Conversely, 'chronic' or 'stable' psoriasis implies the lesions have not significantly changed for months or even years. Clinically active disease presents as new small pinpoint lesions which enlarge to form plaques. In addition, existing plaques increase in size and may join to form large confluent areas of involvement. If the disease is very active then erythrodermic psoriasis will result.

When the disease is inactive the lesions will resolve to leave normal-looking skin, although sometimes there is hypopigmentation, but this is not permanent. When a lesion resolves it may clear from the centre of the plaque, before the periphery, giving rise to an annular lesion. Alternatively the lesion resolves uniformly.

As a general rule when the disease is active all existing lesions are enlarging, and when the disease is inactive all or most of the lesions will resolve, again implying a uniformity in the disease. Active disease implies a poor prognosis, certainly for the immediate future. When the disease is active then whatever treatment is employed to clear the disease there will be a rapid recurrence, and maintenance treatment will be necessary to keep the patient clear. If the disease shows signs of stability, however, the relapse rate after treatment, whatever modality is used, will be low. Therefore it is important to use the clinical signs of disease activity to decide on treatment and give the patient a prognosis at least for the immediate future.

The factors which influence disease activity are at present unknown. Certainly the known triggers discussed above may transform chronic into active disease, but in the majority of patients no external exacerbating factor is discernible. There is now accumulating evidence for both humoral and cellular factors in the initiation and maintenance of lesions, but these appear to be under some form of central control. However, from the clinical point of view it must be emphasized that disease activity may vary in time, and that chronic disease will

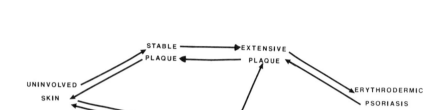

Figure 1.12   Degree of activity of psoriasis and clinical expression

pass into an active phase and vice-versa (Figure 1.12). Patients may remain in an active phase for many years or even indefinitely, and these are the patients whose disease is difficult to control and who require long-term maintenance (usually systemic) treatment. Conversely, patients may go into remission after many years of either chronic or active disease. As yet there are no treatments which will convert active into chronic disease or full remission state.

COMPLICATIONS

These are very rare, and are usually seen only in patients with erythroderma or generalized pustular psoriasis. The majority of patients with psoriasis have no physical complications.

Complications of severe psoriasis
● Infection
● Hypothermia
● Hyperthermia
● Oedema
● Cardiovascular
● Anaemia
● Hypoalbuminaemia
● Hair loss

Infection

Secondary bacterial infection of psoriasis is uncommon, although 50% of patients carry *Staphylococcus aureus* in their lesions. Psoriatic lesions have a very good blood supply, and this may enable them to deal with bacterial infections. In generalized pustular psoriasis, however, when patients are severely ill they appear more prone to skin staphylococcal infections and septicaemia.

Fungal infections in the groins in intertriginous psoriasis are common, and fairly resistant to treatment. This may be due to the long-term use of topical corticosteroids at these sites. There appears to be no increased incidence of viral infections.

Liver Disorders

Minor histological changes in the liver architecture, and 'fatty change', have been found in a small proportion of psoriatics in liver biopsies prior to treatment with methotrexate. It has been argued that these findings are secondary to increased alcohol intake, but others have maintained it is a true association with psoriasis. Jaundice has been described in erythrodermic psoriasis due to liver damage, but whether this is due to the disease, or the drugs used to treat the psoriasis, has not been proven.

Hypothermia

In psoriasis there is increased blood flow to the skin and if the disorder is widespread, as in erythrodermic disease, then there will be increased heat loss which can result in hypothermia.

Hyperthermia

If the ambient temperature is high, as in the tropics, hyperthermia may occur in generalized psoriasis. This is due to occlusion of the sweat ducts by the psoriatic epidermis.

Oedema

This is a common sign in widespread psoriasis, particularly of the legs. Ankle oedema is seen in extensive plaque psoriasis as well as the generalized forms of the disease. The oedema results from the increased capillary permeability associated with the inflammatory changes, and from hypoalbuminaemia in generalized psoriasis.

Cardiovascular

Another complication of the increased blood flow through the skin in generalized psoriasis is the possibility of high-output cardiac failure. The increased blood flow through the skin results in hypervolaemia and subsequent increased cardiac output. In the majority of patients with no preceding cardiac disease the altered haemodynamics do not usually cause problems of failure, but in elderly patients with impaired cardiac function heart failure may ensue.

Anaemia

This is seen only in extensive psoriasis, and is usually mild. Hypervolaemia may in part cause a relatively low haemoglobin concentration. In addition there may be iron deficiency due to (a) chronic inflammation, and (b) iron loss in the scales which are shed in increased amount. Folate deficiency may also occur due to increased utilization in the hyperproliferative skin.

Hypoalbuminaemia

This is due partly to (a) increased capillary permeability, (b) hypervolaemia causing haemodilution and (c) a mild protein-losing enteropathy which occurs in extensive and severe skin disease.

Renal Disorder

In acute generalized pustular psoriasis, severe loss of plasma proteins into tissues occurs, and the subsequent oligaemia may cause acute renal tubular necrosis.

Hair Loss

Scalp and body hair is lost in erythrodermic psoriasis. The cause is unknown, but the hair regrows when the skin returns to normal.

DIFFERENTIAL DIAGNOSIS

Plaque Psoriasis

Seborrhoeic eczema may have a similar appearance to psoriasis, but the lesions are not as thick, and the classical sites are different. Seborrhoeic eczema characteristically affects the face (psoriasis is rare on the face) and centre of the chest and back. If seborrhoeic eczema does affect the limbs the diagnosis may be difficult, and a biopsy may have to be considered.

Discrete chronic patches of eczema on the lower legs, so-called lichen simplex, may be as thick as psoriasis and have a scaly surface. However, the scale is not as loose and white on excoriation with a spatula. Lichen simplex is often unilateral whilst psoriasis is usually bilateral. Skin markings are often intensified in eczema but lost in psoriasis.

> **Differential Diagnosis**
> (Plaque psoriasis)
>
> ● Seborrhoeic eczema
> ● Lichen simplex (localized hypertrophic eczema)
> ● Discoid eczema
> ● Hypertrophic lichen planus
> ● Bowen's disease (intra-epidermal carcinoma)
> ● Mycosis fungoides (T-cell lymphoma)
> ● Pityriasis rubra pilaris
> ● Superficial basal cell carcinoma

Hypertrophic lichen planus on the legs may mimic psoriasis, as these lesions often have a scaly surface, and may be symmetrical. Lichen planus usually has a violaceous rather than a red colour as seen in psoriasis. The more classical lesions of lichen planus elsewhere on the body and in the mouth may be present and confirm the diagnosis. A biopsy will distinguish between the two conditions.

Bowen's disease (intra-epidermal carcinoma) presents as a well-demarcated and scaly patch. It is usually a solitary lesion, and if more than one lesion is present these are asymmetrical. The scales are more adherent, and if removed by scraping with a spatula, pinpoint capillary bleeding points are not seen. The commonest site for Bowen's disease is on the lower leg, whereas psoriasis is most frequently seen on the knees. A biopsy is necessary if Bowen's disease is suspected.

Discoid eczema presents as a symmetrical eruption on the limbs, but the lesions are often crusted rather than scaly. In eczema there tends not to be a sharp line of demarcation between involved and uninvolved skin as seen in psoriasis.

Mycosis fungoides (a cutaneous T-lymphocyte lymphoma) may present as discrete red scaly patches. However, mycosis fungoides is not usually as symmetrical as psoriasis, the scaling is not as 'loose' and capillary bleeding is not present on 'grattage'. If there is any doubt as to the diagnosis a biopsy is necessary.

Pityriasis rubra pilaris is a rare disorder with lesions which may have a similar appearance to psoriasis. The distinguishing features are follicular papules, particularly on the dorsa of the fingers, and yellow hyperkeratosis on the palms and soles.

Superficial basal cell carcinoma is usually found on the trunk as a discrete solitary patch. Occasionally multiple asymmetrical lesions are present due to arsenic medication in the past. The lesion has a red, scaly or crusted surface, and on close inspection a raised pearly edge is visible. Biopsy will confirm the diagnosis.

Guttate Psoriasis

Pityriasis rosea, like guttate psoriasis, tends to appear suddenly, and predominantly on the trunk. Pityriasis rosea may have a herald patch, a discoid or annular lesion which appears about a week before the generalized rash. Classically pityriasis rosea has oval lesions, with the long axis in the lines of the intercostal nerves, and fine centripetal scaling is present, rather than the white scaling seen in psoriasis.

Secondary syphilis may present as a widespread papular eruption. In syphilis there is often involvement of the face, palms and soles. If there is any clinical suspicion of syphilis it is important to do serology tests.

Differential diagnosis
(guttate psoriasis)

● Pityriasis rosea
● Secondary syphilis
● Drug eruptions
● Pityriasis lichenoides – chronic

Pityriasis lichenoides chronica is a rare disease which has small scaly red papules. The scaling is different from psoriasis, in that there is a discrete central scale which peels off in one place, rather than the flaking seen in psoriasis. Pityriasis lichenoides tends to be more widespread with involvement of the limbs as well as the trunk, and as the name implies is a chronic persistent rash rather than one which clears after 3–4 months.

Drug eruptions which usually have a sudden onset like guttate psoriasis, tend not to be as scaling as psoriatic lesions. Gold may give rise to scaly patches, and the history of drug intake should suggest the diagnosis.

Flexural or Intertriginous Psoriasis

Seborrhoeic eczema, like psoriasis, tends to involve the intertriginous areas. Psoriasis lesions tend to be thicker and have a more sharply defined edge than eczematous ones. The distinction between the two disorders can be difficult if there are no lesions on the non-intertriginous skin.

Ringworm fungal infections are predominantly seen in the groins and advance from the intertriginous area. A raised scaly edge with clearing in the central part of the lesion suggests the diagnosis of a fungal infection. In *Candida albicans* infection satellite papules or pustules are present.

Erythrasma, a bacterial infection due to *Corynebacterium minutissimum,* is found in intertriginous areas; it tends to be less thick than psoriasis and have a reddish-brown colour. The diagnosis can be confirmed by finding the organism on skin scrapings, or irradiation with a Woods lamp (ultraviolet light) gives a pink fluorescence.

Genitalia

Penile lesions of psoriasis have to be distinguished from seborrhoeic eczema. The lesions often have a similar appearance in both diseases, although in psoriasis they may be more discrete. If there are lesions elsewhere this should establish the diagnosis. Erythroplasia of Queyrat (intra-epidermal carcinoma) may present as a solitary shiny plaque on the glans penis. If there is doubt as to the diagnosis a biopsy is necessary.

Palm and Sole Psoriasis

There are two types of psoriasis at these sites, the confluent red scaly plaque disease and localized pustular psoriasis. The plaque disease has to be distinguished from chronic hand eczema. Both disorders may show severe hyperkeratosis with fissuring. There may be a history of blisters in eczema. Once again the distinguishing feature may be the sharp cut-off point between the involved and uninvolved skin which is seen in psoriasis but less commonly in eczema. Lichen planus of the palms and soles may also give rise to hyperkeratotic plaques, but the more typical lesions of lichen planus are usually present at other sites.

Localized pustular psoriasis has to be distinguished from secondarily infected eczema. The history and bacteriological examination will usually distinguish the two diseases.

Erythrodermic Psoriasis

Erythroderma may also be due to eczema, cutaneous lymphoma, or be drug-induced. The appearances are similar whatever the aetiology. The history may well indicate the underlying cause, and a biopsy is necessary to exclude or substantiate a lymphoma.

Generalized Pustular Psoriasis

The disease most likely to be confused with generalized pustular psoriasis is subcorneal pustular dermatosis, another rare disease. Constitutional upset and a previous history of psoriasis are likely in pustular psoriasis.

Scalp Psoriasis

When psoriasis only involves the scalp it may be difficult to distinguish from seborrhoeic eczema at this site. The plaques in psoriasis are generally more discrete and thicker, and involvement at the hair line may show the typical white scale. Capillary bleeding points on 'grattage' may occur in both disorders. Hair loss is rare in both disorders but is more likely in psoriasis.

Nails

Pits in the nails are not exclusive to psoriasis, and have been reported in eczema, lichen planus and alopecia areata. In eczema and lichen planus it is usual to see disease of the nail fold, and the hair abnormality will give the diagnosis in alopecia areata.

Onycholysis is not an infrequent occurrence when no skin lesions are present, particularly in females. The question has always been asked whether this abnormality is due to underlying psoriasis or whether there is another cause. As yet there is no satisfactory way to determine if the onycholysis is idiopathic or due to psoriasis. Onycholysis may be seen in ringworm fungal infections of the nail. However, in psoriasis the onycholysis is frequently the only nail abnormality, whereas in fungal infections there are other abnormalities present, e.g. dystrophy and subungual hyperkeratosis.

Subungual hyperkeratosis and dystrophy has to be distinguished from ringworm fungal infection of the nail plate. The latter is more commonly seen in the toe nails, whereas psoriasis affects finger nails more frequently. In psoriasis either all the finger nails or only some of them may be affected, whereas in fungal infections it is rare to see all the finger nails involved. The only certain way of distinguishing between the two conditions is by taking specimens of the nail for mycological examination.

THE UNINVOLVED SKIN

Although the uninvolved skin in psoriatic subjects looks normal, abnormalities have been found, and it would seem that psoriasis is a generalized skin disorder, but what determines clinical expression of the disease remains to be elucidated. In the clinically uninvolved dermis there is a lymphocytic infiltrate similar to that of the involved skin. This would seem to imply that the skin everywhere is prepared to develop into a lesion, and all that is required is a specific stimulus. This may explain the basis of the Koebner phenomenon in response to injury, although an additional factor is required, as the majority of patients do not exhibit the Koebner phenomenon. It has also been shown that compared to normal skin more basal epidermal cells are synthesizing DNA.

PSORIATIC ARTHROPATHY

An association between psoriasis and an arthritis was mentioned in the early part of the nineteenth century. However, there was no uniform agreement as to whether the arthropathy was part of the rheumatoid arthritis spectrum, or a separate entity. It is only in the past two or three decades that psoriatic arthropathy has been recognized as a separate disorder to rheumatoid arthritis. One of the problems in defining psoriatic arthropathy is whether it may exist without the skin lesions.

If this is accepted then there appears to be significant overlap with ankylosing spondylitis and other spondarthritides. A working definition of psoriatic arthropathy would be 'an inflammatory arthritis either peripheral or with spinal involvement in association with psoriasis, and seronegative for the rheumatoid factor'.

Psoriatic arthropathy:
clinical types

- Asymmetrical oligoarthropathy
- Interphalangeal joints
- Distal interphalangeal joints (only)
- Multiple joints – Similar to rheumatoid arthritis
- Severe mutilating arthropathy
- Peripheral arthropathy with sacroiliitis and/or spondylitis

---

Epidemiology

The incidence of arthropathy in patients with psoriasis has varied from 0.5 to 40% in different studies. This variation probably depends on the criteria used to establish the presence of an arthropathy, or missing the minimal skin involvement which may occur in some individuals. It would appear from the more careful studies that the incidence of an arthropathy in psoriasis is between 5 and 7%[11]. The prevalence of arthritis in non-psoriatic dermatological patients has been reported as 0.7%[12].

Investigating the incidence of psoriasis in patients with arthritis has shown a normal incidence for the seropositive, but 4 times normal in patients with seronegative arthritis, supporting the association between psoriasis and arthropathy[13]. The overall incidence of psoriatic arthropathy in the general population has been estimated to be between 0.02 and 0.10%. The sex ratio for psoriatic arthropathy has been shown to be 1:1.39, M:F, compared to 1:3 for rheumatoid arthritis.

Genetics

As with skin lesions there is evidence to support a genetic mechanism in psoriatic arthropathy. Family studies have shown clustering, but no clear Mendelian pattern of inheritance has emerged. It appears that genetic transmission, as for the skin lesions, is based on multifactorial inheritance with environmental factors playing an important part in triggering arthritis.

An increased incidence of HLA-B27 (95%) is now recognized in ankylosing spondylitis. This antigen has also been found to be raised in psoriatic arthritis if there is spinal involvement[14], the incidence being 80% for spinal involvement but 20% for peripheral arthritis. Other HLA antigens, A26, B38 and DR4, have been found to be raised in peripheral arthropathy.

Clinical Features in Peripheral Arthropathy

There are five groups of psoriatic arthropathy which have been outlined.

(1) The most common presentation is mono- or asymmetrical oligoarthropathy. This usually affects the interphalangeal joints, either the distal or proximal.

(2) Exclusive involvement of the distal interphalangeal joints of the toes or fingers. Involvement of these joints is said to be characteristic of psoriatic arthropathy, and dis-

tinguishes it from rheumatoid arthritis, which does not affect these joints.

(3) The presentation which is indistinguishable from rheumatoid arthritis, but the psoriatic disease runs a more benign course.

(4) A severe mutilating arthritis, as seen in rheumatoid disease, but with involvement of the distal interphalangeal joints.

(5) A peripheral arthropathy associated with sacroiliitis and/or spondylitis.

The incidence of the common oligo-arthropathy has been found to be 50% of the psoriatic arthropathies. The severe mutilating form and localization to the distal interphalangeal joints are 8% each.

Thirty per cent of all psoriatic patients with arthropathy have spondylitis.

The peak age of onset for psoriatic arthropathy is between 35 and 45 years. The severe mutilating form usually begins earlier. The onset is acute in approximately 50% of patients. The skin and joint lesions do not usually commence at the same time, but nail dystrophy and joint involvement often appear together.

Spinal Arthritis

There is now a recognized association between psoriasis and sacroiliitis and/or ankylosing spondylitis. The arthropathy may involve the sacroiliac joints and spine together or separately. It is most common for both to be involved.

Relationship between Skin Lesions and Arthropathy

The skin lesions first appear in the majority of patients, only 16% beginning with joint problems. In the latter group, those patients would be termed as having seronegative arthritis, until such as they may develop the rash. It does appear that there may be a small group with classical features of psoriatic arthropathy, i.e. distal interphalangeal involvement, who do not go on to develop psoriasis.

There is a strong association between generalized pustular psoriasis and arthritis, 30% of these patients have an arthropathy.

It has been found in some surveys that the more extensive the psoriasis the more likely the arthropathy.

Relationship between Nail Involvement and Arthropathy

There is a stronger association between joint involvement and nail abnormality than with skin lesions. It has been found that 85% of patients with arthropathy have nail involvement. The nail and joint problems often begin together. No particular one of the varying nail abnormalities is associated with the arthropathy.

Extra-articular Features

These have a lower incidence than those of rheumatoid arthritis. Subcutaneous nodules and involvement of the lung, heart or blood vessels do not occur. Ocular involvement has been reported, mainly uveitis and conjunctivitis. Episcleritis is rare.

Ankylosing spondylitis and inflammatory bowel disease have an increased incidence in patients with psoriatic arthritis.

Treatment

In its mildest forms no specific treatment is necessary. The drug therapy of the arthritis is the same as that for rheumatoid arthritis. Non-steroidal anti-inflammatory drugs (NSAIDs) will control a large proportion of patients. In a small number of patients the NSAIDs do appear to make the rash worse, but there is no way of predicting in whom this may occur.

Other drugs which have been found to be helpful in severe disease are methotrexate, cyclosporin, azathioprine and gold salts. All have potential serious side-effects, and patients will have to be monitored closely. There are reports of improvement of the joints when the rash is treated with PUVA.

Drugs to be avoided are antimalarials and systemic steroids. The former have been reported to make the rash worse, and with the latter there may be a flare-up of the rash when the dose of steroids is reduced.

Surgical procedures as for rheumatoid arthritis should be considered if there is severe deformity.

Prognosis

The prognosis in psoriatic arthropathy appears to be better than in rheumatoid arthritis. There is generally less pain and disability. In a 10-year follow-up a third of the patients lost no time from work and 97% had less than 12 months absenteeism[15]. Radiologically there is little deterioration in the majority of patients. Most of the reported fatalities in psoriatic arthropathy have been attributable to the drugs employed, but there is a small risk of amyloidosis.

REFERENCES

1. Hellgren, L. (1967). *Psoriasis: the prevalence in sex, age, and occupational groups in total population in Sweden.* (Stockholm: Almquist & Wiksell)

2. Farber, E., Bright, R. and Nall, N. (1968). Psoriasis: a questionnaire survey of 2144 patients. *Arch. Dermatol.*, **98**, 248–259.
3. Hoede, K. (1957). Ubersichten: Zur Frage der Erblichkeit der Psoriasis. *Hautarzt*, **8**, 433–438.
4. Bandrup, F., Hauge, M., Henningsen, K. and Eriksen, B. (1978). A study of psoriasis in an unselected series of twins. *Arch. Dermatol.*, **114**, 874–878.
5. Svejgaard, A., Nielsen, L., Svejgaard, E., Kissineyer-Nielsen, F., Hjortshoj, A. and Zachariae, H. (1974). HLA in psoriasis vulgaris and in pustular psoriasis – population and family studies. *Br. J. Dermatol.*, **91**, 145–153.
6. Tiilikainen, A., Lassus, A., Karvonen, J., Vartiainen, P. and Julin, M. (1980). Psoriasis and HLA-CW6. *Br. J. Dermatol.*, **102**, 179–184.
7. Karvonen, J. (1975). HLA antigens in psoriasis with special reference to the clinical type, age of onset, exacerbations after respiratory infections and occurrence of arthritis. *Ann. Clin. Res.*, **7**, 301–311.
8. Enfors, W. and Mollin, L. (1971). Pustulosis palmaris et plantaris. *Acta Derm-Venereol.*, **51**, 289–294.
9. Farber, E. M. and Nall, M. L. (1974). The natural history of psoriasis in 5600 patients. *Dermatologica*, **91**, 1–18.
10. Ryan, T. J. and Baker, H. (1971). The prognosis of generalised pustular psoriasis. *Br. J. Dermatol.*, **85**, 407–411.
11. Leczinsky, C. G. (1948). The incidence of arthropathy in a ten year series of psoriasis cases. *Acta Derm-Venereol.*, **28**, 483–487.
12. Hellgren, L. (1969). Association between rheumatoid arthritis and psoriasis in total populations. *Acta Rheumatol. Scand.*, **15**, 316–326.
13. Baker, H. (1966). Epidemiological aspects of psoriasis and arthritis. *Br. J. Dermatol.*, **78**, 249–261.
14. Brewerton, D. A., Caffrey, M., Nicholls, A., Walters, D. and James, D. C. O. (1974). HLA-B27 and arthropathies associated with ulcerative colitis and psoriasis. *Lancet*, **1**, 956–957.
15. Roberts, M. E. T., Wright, V., Hill, A. G. S. and Mehtra, A. C. (1976). Psoriatic arthritis: follow up study. *Ann. Rheum. Dis.*, **35**, 206–212.

2

THE TREATMENT OF PSORIASIS

C. E. M. GRIFFITHS

The very nature of psoriasis by way of its propensity for spontaneous relapse and remission makes the management difficult and variable according to circumstance. The essence of success is based on the forging and maintenance of confidence in the various therapeutic regimes which may be employed. Constant reassurance and an optimistic outlook are required to ensure compliance. The treatment needs show considerable individual variation, and are often a subjective phenomenon. Extensive skin involvement may be regarded with apparent unconcern by some patients, whilst someone dependent on 'image' for a livelihood, such as a photographic model, may be unduly distressed by only one or two plaques of psoriasis.

From the outset the nature of the disease should be explained and questions fully answered, including the all-pervading one 'why have I got it?' As stress, either in mental or physical form, is a known precipitating or exacerbating factor some authorities[1] advocate psychological counselling and in-depth interviews to encourage an understanding and acceptance of underlying problems. A period of rest, in the form of a holiday, away from the environmental pressures which have compounded the problem, is often of benefit.

Nowadays patients are very likely to ask about allergic precipitants of their disease, and as to whether a diet would be beneficial. There is no evidence that allergy as such plays a role; general good health is important but diets play no part[2] in the management and many diets have been tried in the past. Skin disease is always linked in the minds of most patients with contagion and the risk of infectivity. Even if not directly asked the patient should be aware that psoriasis is not an infectious process. Any chronic disease brings with it the fear of malignancy and the non-neoplastic nature of psoriasis should be emphasized.

How then should the psoriasis patient be managed on a more definitive and therapeutic basis? The varying forms of psoriasis require different treatment, as does psoriasis in different anatomical sites. In the majority of cases therapy is along topical lines in both the primary and secondary care situation. Whichever treatments are instigated a decision needs to be made as to whether remission can be achieved with a short course of treatment or whether maintenance therapy is required. Of course there are no hard-and-fast rules, only guidelines; and each case should be judged on its merits. The forms of treatment which will be discussed need not be employed in isolation and many different permutations are available, some of which display definite synergism.

TOPICAL

Tar

The precise mechanisms of this form of therapy have not been elucidated, although for many years wood and coal tar distillates have been the mainstay of topical treatment for psoriasis[3]. Crude coal tar is the product of destructive distillation of bituminous coal and is a mixture of approximately 10 000 different compounds including benzene, naphthalene,

Initial, topical

- Topical cortico-
  steroids.
- Tar.
- Dithranol
- ± Ultraviolet-B.

Secondary, systemic

- Etretinate alone.
- PUVA alone.
- Etretinate + PUVA.

Tertiary, systemic

- Methotrexate.
- Cyclosporin-A.
- 5-Hydroxyurea.
- Azathioprine.

phenols and pitch[4]. The composition of crude coal tar is variable and dependent on the distillation process employed.

Tar on its own has a definite but modest therapeutic effect in psoriasis[5] although is probably best utilized in combination with ultraviolet light as part of the Goeckerman regime.

Following a warm bath and scrubbing the lesions with a soft nail-brush the skin is dried and coal tar and salicylic acid BPC (2% coal tar and 2% salicylic acid) is applied to the plaques prior to covering with tubegauze; an initial concentration of 2–5% crude coal tar is recommended and repeated daily.

The Goeckerman regime has many variations and is preferable to the use of coal tar alone in that it is more efficient in inducing clearing of psoriasis. It is probably best performed as an inpatient procedure. The patient soaks in a warm bath to which has been added Liquor picis carbonis or a proprietary equivalent such as Polytar emollient; as before, the plaques are scrubbed with a soft nail-brush and the skin dried. Whole-body exposure to ultraviolet light follows at a sub-erythema dose prior to application of crude coal tar to the lesions. Again the initial strength of coal tar should be of the order of 2–5% gradually increasing to 10% if necessary. This process is repeated on a daily basis with a gradual increase in ultraviolet light exposure. Using this modified Goeckerman regime clearance may be expected in 3–6 weeks.

Despite the seeming rationale for this form of treatment tar photosensitization is unlikely to play a part as its action spectrum lies in the UVA range and erythemogenesis is almost entirely due to UVB if the light source is a quartz lamp. Interestingly Le Vine et al.[3] found that if the ultraviolet light was given in erythemogenic doses tar was no better than an emollient such as white soft paraffin.

Despite the fears expressed over its safety there is no evidence[6], apart from a few case reports, that there is an increased risk of carcinogenicity following the use of tar. Only one study has shown an increase in cutaneous malignancy[7], and then only with high exposure to the substance.

The main drawback from which tar suffers is that it is not cosmetically pleasing (thereby reducing patient compliance) and unfortunately refining reduces its already fairly moderate potency. Irritation is unusual unless used in erythrodermic or generalized pustular psoriasis; folliculitis occurs commonly.

Tar preparations are used in many different bases, and shampoo and detergent forms are popular for the scalp.

The scalp can also be treated with mixtures of coal tar and keratolytics applied at night to the scalp plaques and shampooed out in the morning. A commonly used mixture is Unguentum cocois co., composed of liquid coal tar 10%; sulphur 5%; salicylic acid 5%; coconut oil 40% and emulsifying ointment 40%.

Dithranol

Dithranol, 1,8-dihydroxy-9,anthrone, is an unstable compound synthesized from anthrone, which is chemically similar to chrysarobin, a naturally occurring substance extracted from tree bark and the name given to Goa powder[8] used in the treatment of fungal skin infections. It was first used as a treatment for psoriasis by Unna in 1916[9] and has now found a place amongst the most widely prescribed therapeutic agents in psoriasis.

Dithranol is usually used as a paste, the best being Lassar's paste comprising zinc oxide, petrolatum and starch, to which is added salicylic acid as an antioxidant preservative. In the standard form of daily dithranol therapy, after a tar bath the paste is applied daily to the plaques using a wooden spatula, beginning with a concentration of 0.1% or 0.05% in the case of type 1 or fair skin (see Table 2.1) as the irritant effect of dithranol is heightened in this skin type[10]. Extreme care should be taken to ensure that the dithranol is applied only to the plaques and not the uninvolved skin, as the irritancy of dithranol will induce burning. Dithranol stains the uninvolved skin, and any clothing which comes into contact with it; the orange-yellow anthroquinine turns purple in an alkaline environment probably as a result of oxidation products[11]. Recent work has shown that this can be removed by 1% potassium hydroxide and Teepol[12]. The dithranol is left on the skin for 23 hours and washed off in a warm bath containing Liquor Picis Carb or equivalent. If no irritation or burning is apparent the concentration can gradually be increased, usually to a maximum of 0.5% or 1%. Successful treatment is apparent by flattening of the psoriatic plaques, and clearance is defined as impalpability of the plaques. This is usually achieved after approximately 3 weeks treatment. The residual dithranol staining of the skin will disappear spontaneously after 1 week.

The face, scalp, genitalia and flexures should not be treated with dithranol, although some authorities[1] prescribe dithranol

Table 2.1   Topical steroid preparations and potency (percentages)

Group I: Mild	
Hydrocortisone acetate	0.10–2.5
Methylprednisolone	0.025
Group II: Moderately potent	
Clobetasone butyrate	0.05
Dexamethasone	0.01
Flumethasone pivalate	0.025
Fluocinolone acetonide	0.01 or 0.006252
Flurandrenalone	0.0125
Desoxymethasone	0.05
Group III: Potent	
Beclomethasone dipropionate	0.025
Betamethasone valerate	0.10
Desonide	0.05
Diflucortolone valerate	0.10
Flucortolone acetonide	0.025
Fluocinolone acetonide	0.025
Fluocinonide	0.05
Triamcinolone acetonide	0.10
Desoxymethasone	0.25
Group IV: Very potent	
Clobetasol propionate	0.05
Diflucortolone valerate	0.30
Halcinonide	0.10

creams for these sites. Standard 24-hour dithranol therapy is ideally performed as an inpatient procedure, and can be modified to include ultraviolet light exposure as described by Ingram[13].

From the unsuitability of 24-hour dithranol therapy to outpatient management have burgeoned the popular short-contact dithranol regimes. This concept was introduced by Shaefer[14] on the premise that dithranol more easily penetrates parakeratotic as opposed to orthokeratotic stratum corneum, and thus need only be applied for short periods of time to achieve the desired effect. Treatment is initiated with 1% dithranol made up in either Lassar's paste or as one of the proprietary wax sticks and gels. Daily application is to the psoriatic plaques alone with care being taken to avoid the normal skin. Dithranol is left in contact with the skin for a period of 30 minutes before removal, although a 10-minute period has been used. If no irritation has occurred 48 hours after the first application the concentration can be gradually increased to a maximum of 3%; 3% dithranol can be used as a maintenance therapy but if treatment has ceased for more than 3 weeks resumption should be at a lower concentration[15].

The irritation of dithranol can be dampened by the use of moderate-strength topical corticosteroids. Some patients find cream or ointment preparations of dithranol more convenient than pastes. Allergic contact dermatitis to dithranol is rarely seen.

How does dithranol exert its therapeutic effect? To some extent this can be explained by the generation of free radicals[16], although in conjunction with increased levels of prostaglandin E_2 these are probably responsible for the irritation seen in dithranol-induced erythema[17]. Inhibition of mitochondrial function has been implicated[18]. Fry and McMinn[19] demonstrated an inhibitory effect on epidermal DNA synthesis. The work of Baker et al.[20] has shown a decline in the numbers of T-helper lymphocytes in the psoriatic epidermis during treatment with dithranol.

Corticosteroids

The advent of potent topical preparations of corticosteroids in the 1960s revolutionized the outpatient treatment of chronic plaque psoriasis. Although the initial enthusiasm has waned somewhat due to side-effects resulting from indiscriminate use, corticosteroids hold an established place in the treatment of psoriasis. They are easy to use, non-irritant and non-staining, unlike tar or dithranol.

As plaques of psoriasis are markedly indurated only potent or very potent corticosteroids (Table 2.1) are of benefit, applied twice or thrice daily for a maximum of 2 weeks. Ointment, as opposed to cream, bases are preferable in view of the scaling so characteristic of psoriasis. The scalp, face, ears and flexures are best treated with corticosteroids as dithranol is too irritant for these sites. To achieve quicker alleviation of infiltrated plaques salicylic acid may be added to the cream or ointment to a concentration of 10%. For the scalp gels or lotions are available. Occlusions under polythene ('Cling-Film' is ideal) should be used with care, as the absorption of steroid is greatly enhanced, particularly if large surface areas are occluded. Combination of topical corticosteroids with other therapeutic modalities is beneficial, and is particularly useful with PUVA or UVB, and to decrease the irritancy of dithranol on adjacent uninvolved skin.

Unfortunately, continued use of topical corticosteroids in an individual often results in the phenomenon of tachy-phylaxis[21] (a slowing-down of responsiveness following repeated application), and relapse of psoriasis appears to occur more quickly after stopping steroid treatment than after other therapies. There are reports of patent preparations pre-cipitating generalized pustular psoriasis[22].

Isolated resistant psoriatic plaques, on the hands for example, may be treated by intralesional injections of steroid, triamcinolone hexacetonide 5 mg/ml[23]. Intralesional steroid may be used either by hypodermic or dermajet injection into the nail fold for psoriatic involvement of the nail.

Side-effects These are seen only if there has been indis-criminate use, and are directly related to site, potency and duration of use. Absorption is greatest from intertriginous areas, and such sites as the face and genitalia where the skin is thin. Systemic absorption is commoner if large areas are treated, though Cushing's syndrome is rarely seen. As a general rule 30 g of ointment or cream should be enough to cover the entire skin surface area. Potent or very potent steroids should never be used for longer than 2 weeks at a time in any site, and not reapplied to that site for at least 6 weeks.

Corticosteroids accelerate the breakdown, and inhibit the formation, of new dermal collagen, thus leading to atrophy and striae. Spontaneous bruising, telangiectasia and masking of cutaneous infection (termed tinea incognito in the case of fungi) are also signs of overuse of topical corticosteroids.

Systemic corticosteroids are rarely indicated in the treatment of psoriasis, although they have been used in the management of generalized pustular psoriasis, erythrodermic and localized pustular psoriasis and psoriatic arthritis. Their use, however, is not to be encouraged.

Corticosteroids slow epidermal cell division[24] and reduce the numbers of psoriatic epidermal dendritic cells and T-helper lymphocytes[20].

PHOTOTHERAPY

PUVA

The term PUVA stands for psoralens + ultraviolet A (UVA). 8-methoxypsoralens (8-mop) are derived from photosensitizing furocoumarins extracted from the fruits of *Anmi majus*[25], an umbelliferous plant of the Nile delta. The photosensitizing potential of 8-mop was first put to dermatological use in 1947[25] for the treatment of vitiligo, and in 1974 Parrish[26] reported the results of oral PUVA in the management of psoriasis. 8-mop absorbs radiant energy in the 210–330 nm range and its greatest photosensitizing effect occurs in the 320–360 nm range (see Table 2.2). Skin photosensitivity to 8-mop is greatest 2–3 hours after ingestion, decreasing significantly after 5 hours. The therapeutic effect is proportional to blood levels. Psoralen is eventually released from treated cells by repair mechanisms.

UVA can induce skin erythema, but the minimal erythema dose is 1000 times that for UVB, which is absorbed in the epidermis whilst 60% of UVA passes through to the upper dermis[27]. UVA also penetrates the human cornea and is

Table 2.2 The electromagnetic spectrum

Light	Wavelength (nm)
Ultraviolet	
UVC	< 290
UVB	290–320
UVA	320–400
Visible	400–700
Infrared	> 700

absorbed by the lens[25]. UVA alone is of no benefit to psoriasis unless prolonged exposures are used.

8-mop is taken orally at a dose of 0.6 mg/kg, as 10 mg tablets, 2 hours before UVA exposure. Occasionally 8-mop induces nausea and this may be alleviated either by reduction in dose, splitting of the dose 3 and 2 hours before UVA, or taking the tablets with food, although this may delay absorption. Irradiation takes place in a PUVA kiosk lined by UVA-emitting fluorescent tubes. The exposure time is dependent on the dose of UVA to be given, which in turn is dictated by the

Table 2.3 Skin type

Skin type	Description
1	Always burn, never tan
2	Always burn then slight tan
3	Sometimes burn, always tan
4	Always tan, never burn
5	Yellow-Brown races
6	Blacks

patient's skin type (see Table 2.3), ideally type 1 skin should not be treated with PUVA. Treatment is repeated three times a week. Depending on response and erythema the exposure time is gradually increased, and clearance should be expected after 5–12 weeks treatment, speed of response depending on skin type. PUVA will clear psoriasis in at least 66% of cases; however, some patients, particularly those whose psoriasis naturally worsens in the summer, may fail to improve, or may even deteriorate. The large European multicentre study[28] recorded a clearance rate of 89% requiring 20 treatments over 37 days with a median UVA dosage of 97 joules. Once clearance or substantial improvement has been achieved most patients benefit from a gradual tailing-down of PUVA before stopping, with maintenance therapy of once a week or once a fortnight treatment continuing for 2 months[29]. On treatment days UVA-opaque goggles or sunglasses should be worn during irradiation, and for the remainder of the day even indoors, as UVA can penetrate window glass, and fluorescent lights emit small amounts of light of this wavelength. Long-sleeved clothing and sunscreens should be used on bright, sunny treatment days.

Contraindications to PUVA therapy are pregnancy (women of childbearing potential should be using a medically approved form of contraception); a past history of cutaneous neoplasm, especially malignant melanoma; the presence of disease exacerbated by light; and a past history of arsenic ingestion or radiotherapy due to their co-carcinogenic effect. In view of the sometimes high temperatures experienced in the PUVA machine, those subjects with a poor cardiovascular status should be carefully assessed prior to embarking on therapy.

Common, though benign, side-effects include erythema 30%, nausea 12%, pruritus 25%[30] and tanning in almost all. Ultraviolet light exposure from any source will accelerate the skin ageing process, and since the introduction of PUVA the main concern for its safety has involved that of cutaneous carcinogenesis. Reshad et al.[31] believed PUVA to be a significant risk factor in the development of non-melanoma skin tumours, but so far no cases of melanoma have definitely been linked to PUVA. The increased incidence of squamous cell carcinoma is even further enhanced in patients previously treated with arsenic, ionizing radiation, or methotrexate[32], skin types 1 and 2[33] and a high cumulative UVA dosage[34]. Other side-effects include 'PUVA lentigines[35]' in up to 53%, although these are rare if the cumulative dose of UVA is less than 100 treatments[36], actinic keratoses varying in incidence from 1.4%[34] to 50%[37]; nail pigmentation may also occur. In view of these effects it is generally agreed that PUVA in the majority of cases should be reserved for those over 45 years of age. There is still some debate as to whether intensive courses or long-term maintenance will ultimately lead to less cumulative UVA exposure. The addition of the vitamin A derivative etretinate to the PUVA regime has been found by most investigators[38] to allow reduction in PUVA dose required to achieve clearance of psoriasis; however, this is not a universal finding. Etretinate is taken orally for a period of 2 weeks prior to starting PUVA; the two treatments then run concurrently.

Topical 8-mop using 0.1–1% lotions or emulsions[39] 5 or 120 minutes prior to irradiation with UVA have been shown to be of benefit for localized psoriasis such as on the palms and soles. There is an increased risk of phototoxic reactions with this method, though.

Psoralen binds to DNA in the presence of UVA and photoproducts formed with pyrimidine bases induce temporary inhibition of DNA, RNA and protein synthesis in epidermal cells, resulting in inhibition of cellular proliferation. PUVA is also responsible for inducing immunological changes in treated subjects, and this is probably the basis of its mode of therapeutic action. There is a decrease in circulating T-helper lymphocytes[40] and an impairment[41] of cutaneous delayed hypersensitivity resulting from a decrease in epidermal Langerhans cells. A reduction in epidermal T-helper cells predates clinical improvement of psoriatic plaques treated by PUVA[42]. Raised serum levels of 25-OH vitamin D have been reported during PUVA therapy[43].

Ultraviolet Light

Natural sunlight is beneficial in the majority of psoriatic patients, although the presence of short- and medium-length UV light increases the likelihood of erythema and burning with indiscriminate exposure, and makes dosimetry difficult. Erythemogenic doses of UVB, wavelength 300–320 nm, are capable of clearing psoriasis and may be given three times per week. This low-intensity selective phototherapy is best used in chronic plaque psoriasis. Commercially available sunbeds and solaria, if emitting UVB and used sensibly, can be of considerable benefit.

The Dead Sea, by virtue of its geographical and geological location (i.e. in Israel and 1000 feet below sea-level) is renowned for its therapeutic value in psoriasis. The constantly evaporating water creates a cloud of water vapour above the sea, thus filtering out the short- and medium-length ultraviolet light and allowing through UVA alone. This, coupled with the undoubted benefits of the chemicals in the Dead Sea, will induce clearance of psoriasis in approximately 4 weeks.

Etretinate

Observations that vitamin A deficiency resulted in xerosis and follicular hyperkeratosis led investigators to believe that supplementation of vitamin A or an analogue would reverse these features if they occurred in skin disorders. Early trials with vitamin A, however, gave disappointing results. Roche synthesized many hundreds of retinal analogues and in the 1970s the synthesis of etretinate signalled an exciting breakthrough in that the ratio of papilloma inhibition to toxicity was very favourable[44].

At present etretinate is only available in an oral form, and prescribing is limited to dermatologists only. In view of its toxicity it is best reserved for severe, recalcitrant, erythrodermic and generalized pustular psoriasis. For severe plaque psoriasis a daily dose of 0.6–0.75 mg/kg is recommended in divided doses. The other approach is to give small doses of 10–20 mg/day and gradually increase, depending on response. If etretinate is given alone, after 3 months treatment 90% of patients will have a greater than 50% clearance of their psoriasis[45]. The decision to use etretinate is easier for erythrodermic and generalized pustular psoriasis, but in the case of chronic plaque one must weigh up the risk-to-benefit ratio. Realistically etretinate is not suitable for those patients with minimal psoriasis who will most likely respond to other safer forms of therapy.

Generalized pustular psoriasis responds dramatically to only a few days etretinate treatment, although maintenance is required. Palmo-plantar, pustular psoriasis responds, but after 4–6 months treatment patients may complain of uncomfortable thinning of the palms and soles. It is debatable whether etretinate is of value in psoriatic arthritis.

If etretinate is combined with PUVA or UVB it is possible to use lower doses of both modalities. Grupper[46] found that institution of retinoid therapy 1–2 weeks prior to PUVA was better than starting the two concurrently, probably as etretinate will reduce scaling and thickness of plaques. If etretinate is combined with either corticosteroids or dithranol lower doses can be used. Etretinate has been used in conjunction with methotrexate[47], and may allow a graduated transition from methotrexate to etretinate therapy.

Side-effects Virtually all the known side-effects of etretinate have been described as part of the hypervitaminosis A syndrome. Peeling of the palms and soles, dryness of lips and mucous membranes and cheilitis are the commonest reported side-effects. Mucous membrane involvement may result in epistaxes and conjunctivitis. A third of patients have an erythematous tinge to their skin, and up to 50% may exhibit 'retinoid dermatitis[48]', in which the skin becomes 'sticky'. Diffuse hair loss is commoner in females; 75% detect some hair loss although objectively this figure is nearer 25%[45]. This effect is dose-related.

Animal studies show an increase in endogenous production and a decrease in degradation and utilization of triglycerides[45]. During etretinate therapy approximately 50% of patients will exceed a serum triglyceride level of 250 mg/dl, and 20% will exceed 300 mg/dl for cholesterol[45]. These changes are reversible on stopping therapy. Those patients who smoke, drink alcohol, are overweight, or have a family history of lipid abnormalities or diabetes mellitus are at the greatest risk from hyperlipidaemia. On this basis fasting serum lipids should be measured before starting etretinate and at regular intervals during the therapeutic period.

Twenty per cent of patients show a change in liver enzymes; in 1% of cases these changes are persistent[45]. A more serious phenomenon is an idiosyncratic, acute, toxic hepatitis[49].

Etretinate is teratogenic, inducing skeletal malformations and meningomyelocele[50]. The seriousness of the malformations necessitates termination of pregnancy if this occurs whilst on treatment. The long half-life of etretinate (84–168 days) – it has been detected in serum 2 years after cessation of therapy – means that adequate contraception should be practised during treatment and for 2 years after. In the USA a pregnancy test is performed prior to treatment and at regular intervals throughout the course.

Etretinate therapy will probably result in hyperostotic changes in most patients, but only after extended treatment periods. The evidence is conflicting at present, as the majority of patients don't have spinal radiographs before therapy and the incidence of unrelated abnormality is unknown. Gerber et al.[51] were unable to demonstrate an increased incidence of hyperostoses in a group of 37 patients, whilst DiGiovanni et al.[52] found extraspinal calcification in 85% of patients on etretinate for an average of 5 years. In order to limit side-effects and cumulative problems it is advisable to break courses of etretinate therapy after 6–9 months and resume 3 months later if necessary – the so called 'drug holiday'.

The exact way in which etretinate works is still unknown, in psoriasis it reduces epidermal cell proliferation in involved and uninvolved skin. Polyamines are involved in the regulation of cell proliferation, and polyamine levels have been shown to be reduced in the skin of etretinate-treated individuals[53]. Ornithine decarboxylase activity is also reduced by etretinate[54], and this is the rate-limiting enzyme in the formation of poly-amines. These changes predate clinical improvement in the psoriatic lesions, suggesting a primary effect. Cell-mediated immune function has been shown to be both inhibited[55] and stimulated by etretinate.

Etretin, which is the metabolic hydrolysate of etretinate, offers promise in that it is efficacious in severe psoriasis but has a half-life of only 2–4 days[56]. There are many analogues in the pipeline and topical preparations are currently being assessed.

Methotrexate

The precursor of methotrexate, aminopterin, was first used in the treatment of psoriasis by Gubner[57] in 1951, and was rapidly superseded by methotrexate itself in the late 1950s. Initial studies on dosage recommended that methotrexate should be given on a daily basis; however, this seemed to potentiate its hepatotoxicity and by 1966 Callaway et al.[58] were recom-mending a once-weekly oral dose of 0.2–0.4 mg/kg in order to reduce the incidence of hepatic side-effects, and this dosage regime is now almost universally accepted. It is prudent to begin therapy at the lower end of the therapeutic range. If the patient is unreliable as far as compliance is concerned then parenteral methotrexate may be given as a once-weekly 0.2–0.4 mg/kg dose. Unfortunately methotrexate does not seem to work topically or intralesionally.

. Prior to therapy haematological and hepatic function should be tested in the form of a full blood count, liver enzymes and a liver biopsy. Care should be taken in assessment of the pre-treatment liver biopsy, as there are reports of up to 11% of untreated psoriatic patients exhibiting hepatic fibrosis and 0.8% cirrhosis[59]. Most probably these changes are the result of concomitant alcohol abuse. Full blood count and liver function should be measured regularly to start with, and liver biopsy should be repeated with a frequency not less than after every cumulative 1.5 g of methotrexate[23]. As there is a risk in performing liver biopsy, other methods of determining hepatic structure without recourse to biopsy have been studied, including ultrasound[60] and radionucleotide scans. At present no satisfactory replacement method has been found.

Methotrexate is usually used on its own, but can be used in combination with corticosteroids when these are being tailed off, and in conjunction with etretinate when therapy is being changed from methotrexate to etretinate.

Side-effects   Hepatic fibrosis and cirrhosis can occur in up to 25%[61]. These conditions are slow to arise but are an indication for a change in treatment. Fibrotic changes do not seem to be related to cumulative dosage although there is synergism between methotrexate and other hepatotoxins such as alcohol[61]. Fatty change and mild hepatic inflammation may probably be ignored, and may only be fluctuant phenomena.

The incidence of malignancy is debatable, although the study by Stern et al.[62] indicated that there was no substantial increase in the risk of non-cutaneous and cutaneous malignancy in psoriatic patients treated with methotrexate. It may be that the incidence is increased if methotrexate is combined with other immunosuppressive treatment such as PUVA.

Cutaneous[63] and mucous membrane ulceration occur, and may be managed either by a reduction in the weekly dose or a change to alternate-week doses.

Leucopenia, thrombocytopenia and macrocytosis all occur, but if stable and not too severe then methotrexate may be continued.

Ideally methotrexate should not be used in the first half of life, and if it is deemed necessary to prescribe it in women of childbearing potential then adequate contraception should be practised during treatment and for 3 months after cessation as the drug is teratogenic.

Nausea and anorexia on the day of taking the drug are occasionally limiting factors.

Protein binding of methotrexate means that high serum levels may be precipitated by concurrent administration of other protein-binding drugs such as aspirin or sulphonamides.

Methotrexate inhibits DNA synthesis by competing as a substrate for dihydrofolate reductase, thereby inhibiting mitotic activity[64]. There is also an inhibition of poly-morphonuclear leukocyte chemotaxis[65].

5-Hydroxy urea

This is an antimetabolite which blocks DNA synthesis by interfering with the enzyme ribonucleotide diphosphate reductase[66] and was first described as being of benefit in the management of psoriasis in 1970[67]. It is not a first-line treatment and should only be used if more established therapy has failed.

The drug is taken on a daily basis at an initial dose of 0.5 g daily, the maximum being 1.5 g daily in divided doses. Response to treatment is often slow, and it may take up to 2 months before improvement is seen.

The most important side-effect is that of marrow toxicity, and necessitates regular full blood counts. A low haemoglobin is usual, as is macrocytosis[66]. There is no hepatotoxicity. Anagen alopecia may occur.

Azathioprine

Azathioprine has been used in the past for the treatment of psoriasis, but is now out of favour in most centres. Du Vivier et al.[68] demonstrated an improvement in 66% of psoriatic patients treated with this drug, but pulmonary fibrosis occurred in 10% of cases.

Following absorption azathioprine is converted to 6-mercaptopurine and via enzyme competition inhibits nucleic acid synthesis.

The recommended dose is 100 mg daily, increasing if necessary to 200 mg after a period of 2 weeks. The commonest limiting side-effect is marrow toxicity, resulting in agranulocytosis necessitating withdrawal of the drug.

Cyclosporin

The fungal metabolite and immunosuppressive agent cyclosporin was first described as being of benefit in psoriasis in 1979 when Mueller and Hermann[69] used the drug for the treatment of arthritis. Amongst the patients treated were four with psoriatic arthritis, and cyclosporin produced clearing of their psoriasis in a matter of days.

Further work[70–72] has confirmed these findings, and in view of the dose-related nephrotoxicity it is encouraging that relatively low doses of the drug, namely 3 mg/kg daily, will produce clearance of severe recalcitrant psoriasis. The place of cyclosporin in the long-term management of psoriasis has yet to be determined, but it seems to be a useful recruit to the armamentarium.

Cyclosporin has no direct inhibitory action on epidermal growth and primarily inhibits the production of interleukin-2 by activated T-helper lymphocytes, thus suppressing the further proliferation of these cells[73].

Side-effects include nephrotoxicity as a result of interstitial fibrosis and tubular atrophy, and hypertension, either secondary to the deterioration in renal function or primary as a result of a direct sympathomimetic effect on peripheral vasculature. Hirsutism occurs in approximately 40% of patients. Nausea and diarrhoea are common but tolerable. Gingival hypertrophy, malaise and tremor have also been reported, albeit in the higher doses used in the organ transplant programmes. The risk of cutaneous malignancy remains to be determined.

During treatment renal and hepatic function should be monitored regularly, and trough levels of cyclosporin measured, as whole blood levels higher than 750 ng/ml are more likely to be associated with nephrotoxicity.

Dialysis

Several case reports have appeared describing the improvement of psoriasis following haemodialysis and peritoneal dialysis; however, there has been conflicting evidence from controlled studies[74,75]. At present the mechanism of dialysis improvement is unknown, although Glinski[76] postulated that the beneficial effect was a result of depletion of activated polymorphonuclear leucocytes with increased amounts of neutral proteinases. This should remain a wholly experimental technique for the treatment of psoriasis.

Surgery

The physical ablation of psoriatic plaques has been reported using a variety of techniques. Kiil et al.[77] treated isolated psoriatic plaques in 24 patients using serial dermatome shaving to the middle of the reticular dermis. Seventeen of the treated subjects had normal skin in these sites up to 3 years later. The carbon dioxide laser[78], argon laser and cryotherapy[79] have also been used with some success.

This form of psoriatic therapy should be regarded as experimental, but may be of use in experienced hands for treating isolated plaques.

REFERENCES

1. Seville, R. and Martin, E. (1981). *Dermatological Nursing and Therapy.* (Oxford: Blackwell Scientific Publications)
2. Champion, R. H. (1986). Psoriasis. *Br. Med. J.,* **292,** 1693–1696
3. Le Vine, M. J., White, H. A. D. and Parrish, J. A. (1979). Components of the Goeckerman regime. *J. Invest. Dermatol.,* **73,** 170–173
4. Rasmussen, J. E. (1978). The crudeness of coal tar. *Prog. Dermatol.,* **12,** 23–29

5. Petrozzi, J. W., Barton, J. O., Kaidberg, K. and Kligman, A. M. (1978). Updating the Goeckerman regimen for psoriasis. *Br. J. Dermatol.*, **98**, 437–444

6. Bickers, D. R. (1981). The carcinogenicity and mutagenicity of therapeutic coal tar – a perspective. *J. Invest. Dermatol.*, **77**, 173–174

7. Stern, R. S., Zierler, S. and Parrish, J. A. (1980). Skin carcinoma in patients with psoriasis treated with topical tar and artificial ultraviolet radiation. *Lancet*, **1**, 732–735

8. Gorsulowsky, D. D., Voorhees, J. J. and Ellis, C. N. (1985). Anthralin therapy for psoriasis – a new look at an old compound. *Arch. Dermatol.*, **121**, 1508–1511

9. Unna, P.G. (1916). Cignolin als Heilmittel der Psoriasis. *Dermatol. Monatsschr.*, **62**, 116–127

10. Maurice, P. D. L. and Greaves, M. W. (1983). Relationship between skin type and erythemal response to anthralin. *Br. J. Dermatol.*, **108**, 337–341

11. Cairns, R. J. and Hall-Smith, P. (1981). *Dermatology – Current Concepts and Practice*, 3rd edn. (London: Butterworths)

12. Lawrence, C. M., Shuster, S., Collins, M. and Bruce, J. M. (1987). Reduction of anthralin inflammation by KOH and Teepol. *Br. J. Dermatol.*, **116**, 171–178

13. Ingram, J. T. (1953). The approach to psoriasis. *Br. Med. J.*, **2**, 591–594

14. Shaefer, H., Farber, E. M., Goldberg, L. and Schalla, W. (1980). Limited application period for dithranol in psoriasis. *Br. J. Dermatol.*, **102**, 571–573

15. Schwarz, T. and Gschnait, F. (1985) Anthralin minute entire skin treatment. *Arch. Dermatol.*, **121**, 1512–1515

16. Finnen, M. J., Lawrence, C. M. and Shuster, S. (1984) Inhibition of dithranol inflammation by free radical scavengers. *Lancet*, **2**, 1129–1130

17. Barr, R. M., Misch, K. J., Hensby, C. N., Mallet, R. I. and Greaves, M. W. (1983). Arachidonic acid and prostaglandin levels in dithranol erythema: time course study. *Br. J. Clin. Pharmacol.*, **16**, 715–717

18. Swanbeck, G. and Lundquist, P. G. (1972). Ultrastructural changes in mitochondria in dithranol treated psoriatic epidermis. *Acta Dermato-Venereol.*, **52**, 94–98

19. Fry, L. and McMinn, R. M. H. (1968). The action of chemotherapeutic agents on psoriatic epidermis. *Br. J. Dermatol.*, **80**, 373–383

20. Baker, B. S., Swain, A. F., Griffiths, C. E. M., Leonard, J. N., Fry, L. and Valdimarsson, H. (1985). The effects of topical treatment with steroids or dithranol on epidermal T lymphocytes and dendritic cells in psoriasis. *Scand. J. Immunol.*, **22**, 471–477

21. Du Vivier, A. and Staughton, R. B. (1975). Tachyphylaxis to the action of topically applied corticosteroids. *Arch. Dermatol.*, **111**, 581–583

22. Baker, H. and Ryan, T. J. (1968). Generalised pustular psoriasis – a clinical and epidemiological study of 104 cases. *Br. J. Dermatol.*, **80**, 771–793

23. Baker, H. (1986) Psoriasis. In: Rook, A., Wilkinson, D. S., Ebling,

F. J. G., Champion, R. H. and Burton, J. L. (eds), *Textbook of Dermatology*. (Oxford: Blackwell Scientific Publications)

24. Goodwin, P. (1976). The effect of corticosteroids on cell turnover in the psoriatic patient: a review. *Br. J. Dermatol.*, **94** (Suppl. 12), 95–100

25. Abel, E. A. and Farber, E. M. (1980). Photochemotherapy. In: Rook, A. and Savin, J. (eds), *Recent Advances in Dermatology*. (Edinburgh: Churchill Livingstone)

26. Parrish, J. A., Fitzpatrick, A. T. B., Tanenbaum, L. and Patlak, M. A. (1974). Photochemotherapy of psoriasis with oral methoxalen and long-wave ultraviolet light. *N. Engl. J. Med.*, **291**, 1207–1211

27. Everett, M. A., Yeangers, E., Sayre, R. M. and Olson, R. L. (1966). Penetration of epidermis by ultraviolet rays. *Photochem. Photobiol.*, **5**, 533–542

28. Henseler, T., Wolff, K., Honigsman, H. and Christophers, E. (1981). Oral 8-methoxypsoralen photochemotherapy for psoriasis. *Lancet*, **1**, 853–857

29. Melski, J. W. and Stern, R. S. (1982). Annual rate of psoralen and UVA treatment of psoriasis after initial clearing. *Arch. Dermatol.*, **118**, 404–408

30. Farber, E. M., Abel, E. A. and Cox, A. J. (1983). Long-term risks of psoralen and UVA therapy for psoriasis. *Arch. Dermatol.*, **119**, 426–431

31. Reshad, H., Challoner, F., Pollock, D. J. and Baker, H. (1984). Cutaneous carcinoma in psoriatic patients treated with PUVA. *Br. J. Dermatol.*, **110**, 299–305

32. Cox, N. H., Jones, S. K., Downey, D. J., Tuyp, E. J., Jay, J. L., Moseley, H. and Mackie, R. M. (1987). Cutaneous and ocular side effects of oral photochemotherapy: results of an 8-year follow-up study. *Br. J. Dermatol.*, **116**, 145–152

33. Stern, R. S., Thibodeau, L. A., Kleinerman, R. A., Parrish, J. A. and Fitzpatrick, T. B. (1979). Risk of cutaneous carcinoma in patients treated with oral methoxsalen photochemotherapy for psoriasis. *N. Engl. J. Med.*, **300**, 809–813

34. Honigsman, H., Wolff, K., Gschnait, F., Brenner, W. and Jaschke, E. (1980). Keratoses and non-melanoma skin tumors in long-term photochemotherapy (PUVA). *J. Am. Acad. Dermatol.*, **3**, 406–414

35. Miller, R. A. (1982). Psoralens and UVA induced stellate hyper-pigmented freckling. *Arch. Dermatol.*, **118**, 619–620

36. Rhodes, A. R., Stern, R. S. and Melski, J. W. (1983). The PUVA lentigo: An analysis of predisposing factors. *J. Invest. Dermatol.*, **81**, 459–463

37. Abel, E. A., Cox, A. J. and Farber, E. M. (1982). Epidermal dystrophy and actinic keratoses in psoriatic patients following oral psoralen photochemotherapy (PUVA). Follow-up study. *J. Am. Acad. Dermatol.*, **7**, 333–340

38. Fritsch, P. O., Honigsman, H. and Wolff, K. (1983). Isoretinoin – PUVA for psoriasis. *Lancet*, **1**, 236

39. Dunno, K., Honio, T., Ozaki, M. and Imamora, S. (1983). Topical 8-methoxypsoralen photochemotherapy of psoriasis: a clinical study. *Br. J. Dermatol.*, **108**, 519–524

40. Moscicki, R. A., Morison, W. L., Parrish, J. A., Block, K. J. and Colvin, R. B. (1982). Reduction of the fraction of circulating helper-inducer T cells identified by monoclonal antibodies in psoriatic patients treated with long term psoralen/ultraviolet A radiation (PUVA). *J. Invest. Dermatol.,* **79**, 205–208

41. Friedmann, P. S. (1981). Disappearance of epidermal Langerhans cells during PUVA therapy. *Br. J. Dermatol.,* **105**, 219–221

42. Baker, B. S., Swain, A. F., Griffiths, C. E. M., Leonard, J. N., Fry, L. and Valdimarsson, H. (1986). Epidermal T lymphocytes and dendritic cells in chronic plaque psoriasis: the effects of PUVA treatment. *Clin. Exp. Immunol.,* **61**, 526–534

43. Shuster, S., Chadwick, L., Moss, C. and Marks, J. (1981). Serum 25-OH vitamin D after photochemotherapy. *Br. J. Dermatol.,* **105**, 421–424

44. Bollag, W. (1983). The development of retinoids in experimental and clinical oncology and dermatology. *J. Am. Acad. Dermatol.,* **9**, 797–805

45. Ellis, C. N. and Voorhees, J. J. (1987). Etretinate therapy. *J. Am. Acad. Dermatol.,* **16**, 267–291

46. Grupper, C. and Berretti, B. (1981). Treatment of psoriasis by oral PUVA therapy combined with aromatic retinoid (Ro 10-9359; Tigason). *Dermatologica,* **162**, 404–413

47. Vanderveen, E. E., Ellis, C. N., Campbell, J. P., Case, P. C. and Voorhees, J. J. (1982). Methotrexate and etretinate as concurrent therapies in severe psoriasis. *Arch. Dermatol.,* **118**, 660–662.

48. Molin, L., Thomsen, K., Volden, G. and Wantzin, G. L. (1985). Retinoid dermatitis mimicking progression in mycosis fungoides: a report from the Scandinavian mycosis fungoides group. *Acta Dermato-Venereol.,* **65**, 69–71

49. Weiss, V. C., West, D. P., Ackerman, R. and Robinson, L. A. (1984). Hepatotoxic reactions in a patient treated with etretinate. *Arch. Dermatol.,* **120**, 104–106

50. Grote, W., Harms, D., Janig, U., Kietzmann, H., Ravens, U. and Schwarze, I. (1985). Malformation of fetus conceived 4 months after termination of maternal etretinate treatment. *Lancet,* **1**, 1276

51. Gerber, L. H., Hefgott, R. K., Gross, E. G. et al. (1984). Vertebral abnormalities associated with synthetic retinoid use. *J. Am. Acad. Dermatol.,* **10**, 817–823

52. DiGiovanna, J. J., Hefgott, R. K., Gerber, L. H. and Peck, G. L. (1986). Extraspinal tendin and ligament calcification associated with long-term therapy with etretinate. *N. Engl. J. Med.,* **315**, 1177–1182

53. Kaplan, R. P., Russell, D. H. and Lowe, N. J. (1983). Etretinate therapy for psoriasis: clinical responses, remission times, epidermal DNA and polyamine responses. *J. Am. Acad. Dermatol.,* **8**, 95–102

54. Lowe, N. J., Kaplan, R. P. and Breeding, J. (1982). Etretinate treatment for psoriasis inhibits epidermal ornithine decarboxylase. *J. Am. Acad. Dermatol.,* **6**, 697–698

55. Soppi, A.-M., Soppi, E., Eskola, J. and Jansen, C. T. (1982). Cell-mediated immunity in Darier's disease: effect of systemic retinoid therapy. *Br. J. Dermatol.,* **106**, 141–152

,56. Kingston, T. P., Matt, L. H. and Lowe, N. J. (1987). Etretin therapy for severe psoriasis. *Arch. Dermatol.*, **123**, 55–58

57. Gubner, R. (1951). Effect of aminopterin on epithelial tissues. *Arch. Dermatol. Syphilol.*, **64**, 688–699

58. Callaway, J. L., McAfee, W. C. and Finlayson, J. R. (1966). Management of psoriasis using methotrexate therapy orally in a single weekly dose. *S. Med. J. Nashville*, **59**, 424

59. Zachariae, H. (1984). Liver. In: Maibach, H. I. and Roenigk, H. H. (eds), *Psoriasis*. (New York: Marcel Dekker)

60. Miller, J. A., Dodds, H. J., Lees, W. R., Anderson, P. N., Levene, G. M., Munn, D. D. and Kirby, J. D. (1983). A comparison of ultrasonography and liver biopsy in the assessment of methotrexate-induced hepatotoxicity in patients with psoriasis. *Br. J. Dermatol.*, **109**, (Suppl. 24), 24

61. Ashton, R. E., Millward-Sadler, G. H. and White, J. E. (1982). Complications in methotrexate treatment of psoriasis with particular reference to liver fibrosis. *J. Invest. Dermatol.*, **79**, 229–232

62. Stern, R. S., Zierler, S. and Parrish, J. A. (1982). Methotrexate used for psoriasis and the risk of non-cutaneous and cutaneous malignancy. *Cancer*, **50**, 869–872

63. Baker, H. (1970). Intermittent high dose oral methotrexate therapy in psoriasis. *Br. J. Dermatol.*, **82**, 65–69

64. Taylor, J. R., Halprin, K. M., Levine, V. and Woodyard, C. (1983). Effects of methotrexate in vitro on epidermal cell proliferation. *Br. J. Dermatol.*, **108**, 45–61

65. Waldsorfer, U., Christophers, E. and Schroder, J.-M. (1983). Methotrexate inhibits polymorphonuclear leucocyte chemotaxis in psoriasis. *Br. J. Dermatol.*, **108**, 45–56

66. Farber, E. M., Pearlman, D. and Abel. E. A. (1976). An appraisal of current systemic therapy for psoriasis. *Arch. Dermatol.*, **112**, 1679–1688

67. Leavell, U. W. and Yarbro, J. W. (1970). Hydroxy urea: a new treatment for psoriasis. *Arch. Dermatol.*, **102**, 144–150

68. Du Vivier, A., Munro, D. D. and Verbov, J. (1974). Treatment of psoriasis with azathioprine. *Br. Med. J.*, **1**, 49–51

69. Mueller, W. and Hermann, B. (1979). Cyclosporin A for psoriasis. *N. Engl. J. Med.*, **301**, 555

70. Van Joost, T. H., Heule, F., Stolz, E. et al. (1986). Short term use of cyclosporin A in severe psoriasis. *Br. J. Dermatol.*, **114**, 615–620

71. Griffiths, C. E. M., Powles, A. V., Leonard, J. N., Baker, B. S., Fry, L. and Valdimarsson, H. (1986). Clearance of psoriasis with low dose cyclosporin. *Br. Med. J.*, **293**, 792–793

72. Ellis, C. N., Gorsulowsky, D. C., Hamilton, E. A., et al. (1986). Cyclosporine improves psoriasis in a double-blind study. *J. Am. Med. Assoc.*, **256**, 3110–3116

73. Bunjes, D., Handt, C., Rollinghoff, M. and Wagner, H. (1981). Cyclosporin A mediates immunosuppression of primary cytotoxic T-cell responses by impairing the release of interleukin-1 and interleukin-2. *Eur. J. Immunol.*, **11**, 657–661

74. Nisserson, A. R., Rapaport, M., Gordon, A. and Nairns, R. G. (1979). Haemodialysis in the treatment of psoriasis. *Ann. Intern. Med.,* **91,** 218–220
75. Anderson, P. C. (1981). Dialysis treatment of psoriasis. *Arch. Dermatol.,* **117,** 67–68
76. Glinski, W., Zarebska, Z., Jablonska, S., Imiela, J. and Nosarzewski, J. (1980). The activity of polymorphonuclear leucocyte neutral proteinases and their inhibitors in patients with psoriasis treated with a continuous peritoneal dialysis. *J. Invest. Dermatol.,* **75,** 481–487
77. Kiil, J., Kiil, J. and Sogaard, H. (1985). Surgical treatment of psoriasis. *Lancet,* **2,** 16–18
78. Bekassy, Z. and Astedt, B. (1985). Laser surgery for psoriasis. *Lancet,* **2,** 725
79. Harrison, P. V., Walker, G. B. and Davies, J. E. (1986). Trauma for psoriasis. *Lancet,* **2,** 1063–1064

3

THE AETIOLOGY AND PATHOGENESIS OF PSORIASIS

B. S. BAKER

INTRODUCTION

The aetiology and pathogenesis of psoriasis remain unknown. Various hypotheses of varying suitability have been put forward in recent years which include suggestions that fibroblasts, capillaries or neutrophils are abnormal in psoriasis, but there is no convincing evidence that any of these abnormalities are of a primary nature. However, there is very strong evidence to support two proposals which are not mutually exclusive; on the contrary they are very compatible. These are firstly that there is a genetic defect of the skin which predisposes it to hyperproliferation, and secondly that psoriasis is a T-cell-mediated disease.

Any hypothesis for the aetiopathogenesis of psoriasis must take into account the various features of the disease (Table 3.1). The clinical features have already been discussed (Chapter 1); the following description will therefore be confined to the cellular characteristics of the psoriatic lesion.

Table 3.1   Characteristic features of psoriasis

Clinical
Spontaneous exacerbations–remissions
Variable Koebner reaction
Restriction by genetic factors
Association with arthritis
Response to immunosuppressive therapy
Phenotypic variability and anatomical selectivity

Cellular
Epidermal hyperproliferation
Abnormal keratinization
Persistent infiltrate of immunocompetent cells
Changes in the capillary bed

HISTOLOGY OF A PSORIATIC PLAQUE

Epidermis

In a fully developed lesion of psoriasis, as best seen at the margin of enlarging plaques[1], the histological picture is characterized by aggregates of neutrophils within the parakeratotic

---

Histology of epidermis

- Presence of microabscesses
- Parakeratosis
- Lack of granular layer
- Thinning of suprapapillary plate
- Regular elongation of the rete ridges with clubbing

---

horny layer (Munro abscesses) (Figure 3.1). The epidermal cells beneath the parakeratotic stratum corneum may also be interspersed with neutrophils forming a small spongiform pustule of Kogoj which is highly diagnostic of psoriasis. The horny layer shows confluent parakeratosis with small foci of

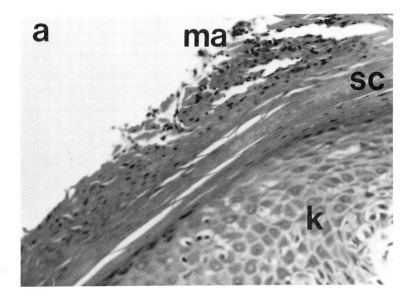

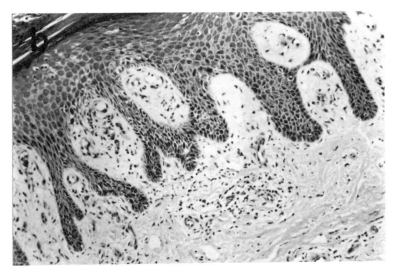

Figure 3.1 Histology of a psoriatic plaque showing: **(a)** aggregates of neutrophils within the parakeratotic stratum corneum; ma = Munro abscess, sc = stratum corneum, k = keratinocytes; **(b)** elongated rete ridges, club-shaped in their lower portion and dermal infiltrate consisting of predominantly lymphocytes and macrophages

orthokeratosis. Since there exists a direct relationship between the absence of keratohyaline granules and the development of parakeratosis, there is widespread absence of stratum granulosum. The stratum malpighii overlying the papillae appears thin. The elongated rete ridges are essentially club-shaped, being narrow in their upper portion but thickened in their lower portion, with neighbouring rete ridges sometimes coalescing at their bases. There is an increase in the number of mitoses, not confined to the basal layer as in normal skin, but extending to two rows of cells above.

Dermis

In the dermis there are changes in the capillary bed which include dilation and tortuosity of the capillaries in the papillary dermis[2], increased capillary permeability[3], enhanced endo-

---

Histology of dermis

- Dilation and tortuosity of capillaries
- Increased capillary permeability
- Enhanced endothelial cell proliferation
- Elevated cutaneous blood flow

---

thelial cell proliferation[4], and elevated cutaneous blood flow[5]. The capillaries are surrounded by an infiltrate of mononuclear cells which extend up into the dermal papillae and are also observed scattered in the epidermis.

EPIDERMAL HYPERPROLIFERATION AND ABNORMAL KERATINIZATION

These features demonstrate a large increase in the numbers of epidermal cells (by a factor of 4 compared to normal skin) together with abnormal keratinization. However, the increased rate of production of epidermal cells in a psoriatic lesion is probably not the result of an altered cell cycle time, as previously believed, but results from two abnormalities; an increase in the absolute size of the germinative compartment, and a much larger proportion of the germinative cells which are actively cycling[6].

Not only the presence of nuclei in the stratum corneum (parakeratosis) but also the absence or substantial decrease of a major component of keratin (α-chain, molecular weight 67 000) in the psoriatic plaque demonstrates an abnormal keratinization process. However, Mansbridge and colleagues[7] suggest that keratinization in the psoriatic lesion progresses via a different pathway from that found in normal skin, rather than by an altered normal pathway.

NATURE OF CELLULAR INFILTRATE

The majority of mononuclear cells in the infiltrate of both early and fully developed psoriatic lesions are T cells and macrophages, with very few B lymphocytes or neutrophils[8,9].

Dermal infiltrate

- Majority are T lymphocytes
  $2 \times T_H > T_S$
  most activated T cells are T_H
  and macrophages
- Very few B lymphocytes
- Very few neutrophils

More recently monoclonal antibodies to human T cell antigens have become available, and this has allowed T cell subpopulations in psoriatic lesions to be studied[10-12]. Monoclonal antibodies are produced by fusing spleen cells from a mouse immunised with human T cells with myeloma cell lines; by repeated subculture and dilution single clones of antibody-secreting cells are established[13]. Staining with Leu 2a (specific for suppressor/cytotoxic T cells) and Leu 3a (specific for helper/inducer T cells) monoclonal antibodies showed that the dermal infiltrate consists of approximately twice as many helper T (T_H) as suppressor T (T_s) cells and that, judged by class II major histocompatibility antigen (HLA-DR) expression, most of the activated T cells are of the T_H subset[12]. Small numbers of T lymphocytes are also present in the epidermis of psoriatic lesions[12]. Unlike normal epidermis in which T lymphocytes are of the suppressor phenotype, the epidermis of pinpoint lesions biopsied within 2 days of their eruption contains moderate numbers of T_H cells, some of which are activated (HLA-DR positive)[12]. These T cells are situated in the basal layer of the epidermis and are mostly in contact with

---

Epidermal infiltrate

Pinpoint lesions
- Moderate numbers of T_H cells
- Some T_H are activated
- Equal numbers of T_S cells
- T_S cells are inactive

Resolving guttate lesions
- $T_S > T_H$
- T_S, but not T_H, cells are activated

Chronic plaques
- $T_S > T_H$
- Equal numbers of activated T_H and T_S cells

HLA-DR positive Langerhans cells (Figure 3.2a, b). The latter are increased in numbers compared to normal skin, and tend to occur in small suprabasal aggregates (Figure 3.2b). Epidermal T_S cells are not increased in these early lesions, and remain inactive as judged by the absence of HLA-DR molecules.

However, in late guttate lesions, which are resolving spontaneously T_S cells again become more prominent than T_H cells (Figure 3.2c, d) and, in contrast to the erupting lesions, nearly all activated T cells are now of the T_S phenotype[12]. This trend was confirmed in sequential biopsies from a single patient with guttate psoriasis in whom fading of the lesions coincided with increasing numbers and the appearance of HLA-DR positive T_S cells[12].

Chronic psoriatic plaques which had remained static in size for at least 1 year show a similar epidermal T_H/T_S ratio to resolving guttate lesions and also markedly increased numbers of Langerhans cells. However, in contrast to the spontaneously resolving lesions, persistent plaques contain approximately equal numbers of activated T_H and T_S cells[14].

AETIOLOGY OF PSORIASIS

The significance of infections, both bacterial and viral, as triggering factors of psoriasis is now well established[15]. The site

---

Aetiology

- Bacterial and viral infections
- Stress
- Drugs
- Hormones
- Physical and chemical trauma

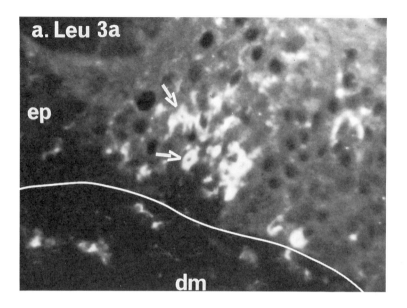

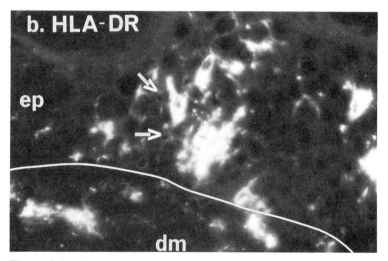

Figure 3.2 Sections of early **(a, b)** and late **(c, d)** guttate psoriatic lesions double-stained with anti-HLA-DR and either Leu 3a or Leu 2a monoclonal antibodies. (Methods described in Ref. 12).

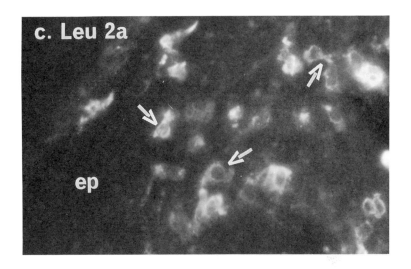

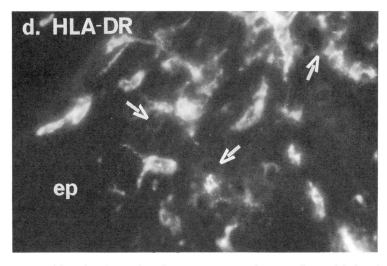

ep = epidermis; dm = dermis; Leu 3a = surface marker of helper/
inducer T cells; Leu 2a = surface marker of suppressor/cytotoxic T
cells. Arrows indicate the position of T cells in consecutive photo-
graphs. Helper (a) and suppressor T cells (c) are seen in close appo-
sition to HLA-DR positive dendritic cells – (b) and (d), respectively

of infection, for example streptococcal[16], is mostly the upper respiratory tract and the clinical picture that of a guttate psoriasis. Stress has also been implicated as a trigger factor in some patients[17]. Other factors that may precipitate or exacerbate psoriasis include drugs such as lithium salts, mepacrine, chloroquine, β-blockers and indomethacin, hormones, and physical and chemical trauma to the skin.

PATHOGENESIS OF PSORIASIS

Location of Primary Defect

The pathogenesis of psoriasis remains to be elucidated. However, most hypotheses which attempt to explain the events which culminate in the formation of a psoriatic lesion are based on the premise that a genetic defect resides either in the skin (epidermis and/or dermis) or in the immune system (cellular and/or non-cellular components).

DEFECT OF THE SKIN

If the skin of patients with psoriasis contains a primary defect there should be evidence that uninvolved skin is also diseased. There is now considerable support for this concept. Abnormalities include increased rates of DNA synthesis[18], enhanced polyamine synthesis[19], plasminogen activator activation[20] and increased levels of free arachidonic acid[21]. DNA synthesis is further abnormally increased after damage to the skin *in vivo*; for example, tape stripping or injection with saline or propranolol[22]. In addition there are increased numbers of both T_H and T_S cells in the dermis of uninvolved psoriatic skin compared to normal dermis, and approximately half of the T_H cells are activated (HLA-DR positive)[12].

To determine whether humoral factors are necessary to maintain the changes in uninvolved skin Krueger et al.[23] compared epidermal proliferation rates of involved and uninvolved skin from patients with psoriasis to normal skin before and after transplantation to congenitally athymic (nude) mice. Nude mice lack T cell function, and are therefore unable to reject grafts of foreign tissue. By definition this system lacks the humoral factors present in the psoriatic host. Before transplantation, both uninvolved and involved psoriatic skin show significantly increased epidermal DNA synthesis compared to normal; 1.6 and 3.6 times, respectively. However, 6 weeks post-transplantation DNA synthesis by epidermal cells of uninvolved skin is increased, and that of involved skin decreased, whilst normal epidermal cell synthesis of DNA is unchanged. These changes are such that involved and uninvolved psoriatic skin acquire equally elevated epidermal cell proliferative activity (2.2 times that of normal skin).

A similar study by Haftek et al.[24] reported preservation of certain immunological identities of grafted skin such as intercellular substance and basement membrane antigens, and an unaltered keratinization pattern throughout the post-grafting period. Furthermore, plasminogen activator, an enzyme found to be increased during cell transformation and activation, is maintained at increased levels in involved psoriatic epidermis, and increases in activity in uninvolved epidermis 6 weeks post-grafting[20]. However, not all features of psoriasis are preserved subsequent to grafting. For example, the granular layer reappeared in involved psoriatic skin grafts as early as 5 days after grafting[24], and polymorphonuclear leukocytes[20] and the abnormal tufting of the capillary network[23] were absent post-grafting.

Thus these findings suggest that there is an inherent defect

Skin

- Inherent defect of epidermal cell proliferation
- Humoral factors involved in disease expression

of epidermal cell proliferation in patients with psoriasis. In addition, host humoral factors (cellular and/or non-cellular) appear to play a role in both expression and non-expression of this disease. Aberrant epidermal cell proliferation may result from a defect in either the epidermis or dermis.

EPIDERMIS

Various biochemical and structural differences have been observed in the epidermis of patients with psoriasis (Table 3.2). However, whether these differences are primary or secondary, or how they relate to the pathogenesis of psoriasis, has not yet been determined. A further interesting observation is that keratinocytes in psoriatic lesions do not frequently express HLA-DR antigens[31], in contrast to those in other inflammatory skin diseases such as lichen planus and contact eczema whose lesions also contain activated T lymphocytes. Activated T lymphocytes synthesize γ-interferon which *in vitro* causes induction of HLA-DR antigen expression on various cell types including keratinocytes[32], and also inhibits keratinocyte cell proliferation[33]. In addition, interferon has no effect on DNA synthesis of psoriatic skin, either when added

Table 3.2   Biochemical and structural differences in the epidermis of patients with psoriasis

1. A 67K keratin polypeptide is absent or greatly decreased in psoriatic scale[25]
2. Increase in size of keratinocytes from both involved and uninvolved skin[26]
3. Increase in number of binding sites for lectins, especially on keratinocytes from involved skin[27]
4. Increase in cohesiveness of the stratum corneum of uninvolved skin[28]
5. Twenty-fold increase in a saturated 23-carbon fatty acid (tricosonic acid) in uninvolved keratinocytes[29]
6. Ten-fold decrease in cholesterol esterase of keratinocytes from uninvolved skin[30]

to cultures in diffusion chambers[34] or when injected directly into psoriatic lesions[35]. These observations suggest that keratinocytes in psoriatic lesions respond abnormally to γ-interferon; this may be of significance with regard to the inherent aberrant proliferation of epidermal cells proposed in this disease.

DERMIS

If hyperkeratotic epidermis (plantar surface) is separated from dermis and then transplanted to dermis in areas that are not usually hyperkeratotic the hyperkeratosis is lost. The converse is also true. These observations suggest that dermis may be important in the differentiation of epidermis, and therefore in the pathogenesis of psoriasis.

Briggaman and Wheeler[36] used recombinant transplantation to investigate the role of dermis in psoriasis. This technique involved removing a thin layer of skin, separating epidermis from dermis, and then recombining it in the various combinations, normal epidermis with dermis from skin involved with psoriasis and vice-versa, then transplanting the recombinants to nude mice. When psoriatic epidermis was recombined with psoriatic dermis an increased labelling index of the same magnitude as that of unseparated specimens was observed. However, the combination of psoriatic dermis and normal epidermis, or of psoriatic epidermis and normal dermis, did not result in an increased labelling index. These findings suggest that both epidermis and dermis are required for the abnormal epidermal cell proliferation observed in this disease. Two possible sites for a primary defect in the dermis are the fibroblasts and capillaries.

Fibroblasts

The role of fibroblasts in the induction of epidermal hyperplasia in psoriasis is somewhat controversial. Baden et al.[37] compared fibroblasts from mice and normal human subjects, and was unable to show that psoriatic fibroblasts were superior in their ability to support epidermal cell growth. Indeed both normal and psoriatic keratinocytes grew better on the mouse fibroblasts than on a feeder layer of psoriatic or normal human fibroblasts, the latter two being equal. In contrast, a skin equivalent model used in a recent study[38] showed that psoriatic fibroblasts *are* able to induce hyperproliferative activity in normal keratinocytes. The skin model consists of a small full-thickness punch biopsy inserted into a dermal equivalent. The dermal equivalent originates from the contraction of a collagen gel by dermal fibroblasts that have been grown as conventional monolayer cultures on plastic. The authors argue that the latter is a better representation of the environment of the actual dermis than the feeder layers used in the previous study, thus explaining the difference in results. However, as both uninvolved and lesional psoriatic fibroblasts are able to induce hyperproliferation of a normal epidermis, other factors must be involved to prevent uninvolved skin becoming lesional. Furthermore, this study excludes the possibility of an inherent defect of the epidermal cells as both normal and uninvolved psoriatic keratinocytes were stimulated by psoriatic fibroblasts.

Capillaries

The possibility that a vascular defect plays a major role in the pathogenesis of psoriasis has long been debated. Morphological studies support this idea with the following observations. The capillary loops in the dermal papillae of psoriatic lesions become dilated and tortuous before overt histological evidence of psoriasis is seen[39]; abnormally dilated capillary loops have been frequently observed in uninvolved psoriatic skin[40]. On the basis of light microscopic studies of developing psoriatic lesions, Pinkus and Mehregan[3] proposed that initial vasodilation accompanied by an exudate of inflammatory cells and serum in the papillae was the initiating event in psoriasis. Several investigators have observed an upward proliferation of the dermal papillae at the edges of developing psoriatic lesions, and believed this to be one of the initiating events of the disease[39].

However, the findings of a more recent study[41] support the concept that the initial stimulus for the epidermal hyper-proliferation in psoriasis resides in the epidermis rather than in the microvasculature. These investigators had previously reported that arterial and venous capillaries could be differentiated by their ultrastructural features[42]. The capillary loops within the dermal papillae of normal skin were shown to be arterial, whereas those of psoriatic skin had the characteristics of venous capillaries. In patients treated successfully with PUVA or the Goeckerman regime, the capillaries began to revert from venous to arterial type 3–8 days before improve-

---

Defect in the skin

Epidermis
- Structural and biochemical alterations of keratinocytes
    ? Significance
- Infrequent HLA-DR expression by keratinocytes
    ?Abnormal response to γ-interferon

Dermis
- Fibroblasts may induce keratinocyte hyperproliferation
- Capillaries probably have a modulatory role

ment in the labelling index of the epidermal cells[41]. However, of the four patients of a total of six who showed clinical improvement, three still had an elevated labelling index even though the loops had returned to normal and the histological features of psoriasis were no longer present. Similarly, in the uninvolved skin of psoriatic patients an elevated labelling index may exist in the presence of both normal histological features and a normal capillary loop configuration. In the light of these observations a modulating rather than primary role has been suggested for the microvasculature in psoriasis.

MOLECULAR NATURE OF SKIN DEFECT IN PSORIASIS

There is therefore strong support for the concept that the primary genetic defect in psoriasis resides in the skin of these patients. The next question to be asked is: What is the nature of this defect? Candidates for this role include intercellular mediators such as cyclic nucleotides, polyamines, arachidonic acid and its metabolites, proteinases and calcium.

Possible site of molecular defect in psoriasis

- Cyclic nucleotides
- Polyamines
- Arachidonic acid and its metabolites
- Proteinases
- Calcium

Cyclic Nucleotides

In 1971 Vorhees and Duell[43] hypothesized that a defective cyclic adenosine monophosphate (cAMP) cascade might explain three characteristics of lesional psoriatic epidermis:

(1) increased proliferation at the basal cell layer,

(2) increased glycogen content of epidermis,
(3) decreased cellular differentiation of the outer portion of
     psoriatic epidermis.

The hypothesis was based on the observation that cAMP could induce breakdown of glycogens and decrease proliferation whilst increasing differentiation.

Epidermal cell metabolism can be influenced by hormone-like molecules such as beta-catecholamines, histamine, adenosine or AMP, prostaglandins of the E series and cholera toxin which, acting through cell surface receptors coupled with the enzyme adenylate cyclase, result in an increase in intracellular cAMP. In psoriatic lesions the ability of beta and prostaglandin receptors to generate cAMP is selectively reduced[44,45]. Furthermore, Iizuka and co-workers[46] have shown that cAMP phosphodiesterase, an enzyme which degrades cAMP to 5'-AMP, is twice as active in psoriatic epidermis, which also could result in a decreased level of cAMP in psoriatic epidermis. However, as discussed by Vorhees[47], the cAMP content of involved psoriatic epidermis has been reported to be higher, the same or lower than uninvolved or normal epidermis. These discrepancies may reflect the multifactorial nature of the disease, or perhaps variability in the activity of lesions at the time of biopsy, or they may result from differences in assay methods.

Cyclic nucleotide pathway changes in psoriatic epidermis

- Defective beta and prostaglandin receptors
- Increased cAMP phosphodiesterase activity
- ? Altered cAMP levels

There is some support for a role in the pathogenesis of psoriasis for a defective cAMP system. For example, lithium, a known inhibitor of adenylate cyclase, induces and exacerbates psoriasis. However, whether this drug directly affects the epidermis or causes an abnormal effect on the immune system that results in clinical expression of disease is unknown[48]. Beta-receptor-blocking agents such as practolol and propranolol will exacerbate pre-existing psoriasis and even induce the development, for the first time, of plaque-type or pustular psoriasis[49]. Indeed, when injected intradermally, propranolol increases the number of proliferating cells in psoriatic epidermis more than in normal skin[22]. On the contrary, agents which inhibit the enzyme breakdown of cAMP, such as papaverine, have been reported to improve psoriasis[50]. However, these drugs have several known mechanisms of action which could account for their effects. Indeed propranolol, in common with lithium, has been shown to affect some immune functions[51].

The other cyclic nucleotide studied in psoriatic epidermis is cyclic guanosine monophosphate (cGMP). Although there is agreement that cGMP levels are elevated in lesional psoriatic epidermis[52,53], the role of cGMP in skin is not clear.

The above findings suggest that a defective cAMP pathway may contribute to the abnormal proliferation of epidermal cells in psoriasis, but there is little convincing evidence that a defect of this kind is of a primary nature.

Polyamines

Polyamines are low molecular weight amines which are essential to cell proliferation. They are present in increased amounts in all actively proliferating cells and have been shown to stimulate RNA and protein synthesis *in vivo*.

Marked abnormalities of the polyamines and their enzymes have been reported in involved (and possibly also uninvolved) psoriatic epidermis[54]. The polyamines putrescine and spermidine, and their biosynthetic enzyme ornithine decarboxylase (ODC), are all elevated in involved skin relative to normal and uninvolved skin. In addition to the epidermis, the urine[54] and the blood[55] of psoriatic patients contain elevated polyamine levels. Clinical improvement of psoriasis by treatment with

---

Polyamines in lesional epidermis
- Putrescine and spermidine increased
- ODC increased

---

steroids, dithranol, retinoids or PUVA is accompanied by a decrease in skin polyamines. In certain tissues, ODC and thus polyamine formation is regulated by cAMP. An inability to inhibit ODC activity due to a defective cAMP cascade may explain the above observations[47]. It is unlikely that these changes in polyamine levels represent a primary defect in psoriatic skin, as similar changes have been observed in several other situations where epidermal hyperproliferation occurs. However, these abnormalities could be involved in the regulation of epidermal growth in this disease.

Arachidonic Acid and its Metabolites

Arachidonic acid (AA) is stored with other polyunsaturated fatty acids in cell membranes where it is bound as phospholipid. Once released, a process catalysed by phospholipase A_2, AA is converted into several different biologically active compounds. This can occur via two different pathways, one involving a cyclic oxygenase and the other lipoxygenases, giving rise to prostaglandins (PGs), 20-carbon, monocarboxylic acids, or to hydroxy-eicosatetraenoic acids (HETEs) and leukotrienes (LTs) respectively.

Although skin, especially epidermis, possesses a high AA-transforming capacity, the cellular origin of the products has not yet been identified.

Several studies have indicated that AA metabolism is misregulated in psoriasis. Both free AA in involved epidermis, and phospholipase A_2 in uninvolved psoriatic epidermis, are increased[56,57]. Increased levels of 12-HETE, PGE_2 and $PGF_{2\alpha}$ have also been reported in psoriatic epidermis[56]; skin chamber

---

AA Metabolites in psoriasis

Lesional epidermis
- Free AA increased
- 12-HETE (and other HETEs) increased
- PGE_2 and $PGF_{2\alpha}$ increased
- LTB_4

Uninvolved epidermis
- phospholipase A_2 increased

---

fluid from abraded psoriatic lesions and extracts of psoriatic scale contain LTB_4 and at least six different HETEs of which 12-HETE is present in highest concentration[58].

The extremely high levels of AA and 12-HETE compared to the more modest elevation of PGE_2 and $PGF_{2\alpha}$ have led to the proposal that the cyclo-oxygenase pathway is inhibited in psoriatic skin[59]. This may divert increased amounts of free AA to the lipoxygenase system whose products may be involved in the pathogenesis of psoriasis. One such product, LTB_4, is the most potent chemotactic agent known and, furthermore, stimulates epidermal proliferation *in vitro*[60]. Other products such as HETEs and LTC_4 are believed to be important mediators of inflammation by virtue of their chemotactic, vasopermeability-increasing and bronchoconstrictive properties[61]. Therefore one might expect that a cyclo-oxygenase inhibitor would exacerbate psoriasis by further increasing the diversion of free AA into the lipoxygenase system. This appears to be the case when indomethacin is applied to psoriatic plaques[62]; conversely the 5-lipoxygenase inhibitor benoxaprofen markedly improves psoriasis[63]. However, it is of interest in this context that PGs of the E series exhibit strong suppressive activity on diverse aspects of the immune response[64].

The AA and cyclic nucleotide pathways are closely linked. AA, HETE and other related intermediates can stimulate cGMP; AA can inhibit the enzyme-forming cAMP, adenylate cyclase[65]. Conversely in other tissues cAMP will inhibit phospholipase A_2 responsible for the cleaving of AA from cell membranes[47]. A defective cAMP-generating pathway could explain the increase in phospholipase A_2 activity in psoriasis. Thus aberrations in the AA metabolic pathway exist in psoriasis. However, although lipoxygenase compounds may be involved in the pathogenic process, their involvement in the primary events of the disease process appears unlikely.

Proteinases

Proteinases are enzymes which degrade the internal backbone of proteins; the serine class proteinases are of primary interest in psoriasis. The serine proteinase plasminogen activator, which converts extracellular plasminogen into the active protease plasmin and is increased in situations in which cell transformation and activation occurs, is dramatically increased in psoriatic plaques[66].

Lazarus et al.[67] have extracted from psoriatic plaque a serine proteinase (? plasminogen activator) that will activate C_5, a possible mechanism for the accumulation of neutrophils in psoriatic epidermis. Of interest in this context are the transplantation studies by Fraki et al.[20], which were discussed earlier. These studies demonstrated that plasminogen activator levels in lesional psoriatic skin remain elevated after transplantation to nude mice, and that uninvolved skin plasminogen activator activity increases to a similar level. Normal skin levels, however, do not change. These observations parallel those of the epidermal labelling index of psoriatic skin after transplantation to the nude mouse[23]. Further studies by this group indicated that plasminogen activator levels in psoriatic skin may correlate with disease activity as measured by extent of skin involvement[68].

Thus there are alterations of proteinase metabolism in psoriatic epidermis which are intrinsic to the skin, do not depend upon circulating factors and which are precise markers of cellular activation. The role of proteolytic enzymes in the pathogenesis of psoriasis is unknown, but they may be involved in the increased epidermal cell turnover and neutrophil accumulation in this disease.

Calcium

Calcium is an essential cofactor of enzyme reactions, and has been shown to be involved in the transition of cells from the proliferative to the differentiated compartment of epidermis. Apart from a report by Vickers and Sneddon[69], who described two patients with hypoparathyroidism in which low serum calcium levels were associated with a flare of the disease, little has been published regarding calcium levels in psoriasis. However, it has recently been reported that the level of the calcium-binding protein calmodulin is specifically and markedly increased in psoriatic lesions[70], and also in clinically uninvolved skin[71]. The significance of these changes in the pathogenesis of psoriasis is unknown.

DEFECT OF THE IMMUNE SYSTEM

Extensive research carried out over the past 20 years has established the involvement of immune mechanisms in the pathogenesis of psoriasis. The linkage between certain histocompatibility (HLA) antigens and psoriasis, the persistence of the disease throughout life once it has manifested itself clinically suggesting the existence of a 'memory', and the spontaneous exacerbations and remissions of disease activity characteristic of diseases involving a chronic immune response are strong supportive evidence for an on-going immune response in psoriasis. Furthermore, effective treatments for psoriasis, such as cyclosporin A, steroids, methotrexate and PUVA, have immunosuppressive activity. Both cellular and non-cellular components of the immune system are implicated in the psoriatic process.

1. Non-cellular Components

Although serum-derived factors are known to participate in cell growth, the involvement of non-cellular humoral factors in the maintenance and resolution of psoriasis has, surprisingly, not been extensively studied. Observations which support the concept that humoral factors are involved in the pathogenesis of psoriasis are:

Transplantation studies The effects of transplanting lesional and uninvolved psoriatic skin onto nude mice have been described previously.

Koebner and reverse Koebner reactions Although poorly understood, it is well documented that localized psoriasis can develop after injury to uninvolved skin of psoriatic patients (Koebner reaction). Some patients who are negative for this reaction also do not redevelop psoriasis in an injured involved site, a phenomenon termed 'reverse Koebner reaction' by Eyre and Krueger[72]. A positive Koebner reaction and a positive reverse Koebner reaction are thus mutually exclusive. Furthermore, all injured areas on a given individual react in a similar manner, supporting the concept that humoral factors are involved in the regulation of disease expression on a body-wide basis.

Effect of psoriatic sera on the Koebner reaction Stankler[73] observed that serum from patients recovering from psoriasis inhibits the Koebner reaction whereas that from patients with active disease does not.

Various abnormalities have been observed in the serum and plasma of patients with psoriasis (Table 3.3). The increases in C-reactive protein and α_2-macroglobulin appear related to severity[74] and, because they are inconsistently present and reflect similar findings in other diseases, are considered insig-

Table 3.3   Serum and plasma abnormalities in psoriasis

1. Increased sedimentation rate, C-reactive protein and α_2-macro-globulins
2. Increased IgA
3. Immune complexes
4. Anti-IgG, IgM and IgA
5. Inhibitor of E-rosette formation
6. Koebner-associated protein
7. Reduced monocyte chemotactic activity
8. Increased angiogenesis-enhancing effect
9. Modulation of endothelial cell proliferation

nificant. An increase in IgA levels appears to be the most prominent immunoglobulin disturbance in psoriasis; most of the immune complexes observed in these patients are of the IgA type[75]. In addition various classes of anti-IgG factors are present in psoriatic sera, as well as bound to the skin and to lymphocytes. In contrast to rheumatoid arthritis in which the anti-IgG (rheumatoid factor) is usually of the IgM class, in psoriasis anti-IgG is of the IgA and IgG classes[76]. The inhibitor of E-rosette formation demonstrated by Glinski et al.[77] in patients with active psoriasis could be an antiglobulin binding to Fc receptors on T lymphocytes[78].

With relevance to the Koebner reaction described above, two-dimensional gel electrophoresis of serum from patients with psoriasis revealed a protein adjacent to GC globulin which is present in 23% of psoriatic patients, but is absent from normal subjects. Furthermore this protein is present in 67% of psoriatic patients with a positive Koebner reaction and only 7% of patients with a negative Koebner reaction[79].

As monocytes from patients with psoriasis have enhanced migratory function to serum, sera from psoriatic and normal individuals were compared as to their effects on monocyte migration[80]. Serum from psoriatic patients was shown to be clearly less chemotactic for monocytes than normal serum; this did not appear to be secondary to excess inhibitors for the chemoattractants. These findings contrast with those demonstrating that serum from patients with psoriasis has enhanced chemotactic activity for neutrophils[81]. Further studies on the effects of psoriatic sera on mononuclear cell function showed that serum from patients with active, rather than static, disease enhanced lymphocyte-induced angiogenesis (new blood vessel formation) in mice[82]. In addition, sera from patients with active psoriasis modulated proliferation of normal human endothelial cells *in vitro*[82]. These findings may be of relevance to the vascular changes, characteristic of new blood vessel formation, observed in psoriatic lesions.

Bound Autoantibodies in Psoriasis

(a) *Stratum corneum antibodies.* Antibodies against stratum corneum occur in essentially all human sera[83], are primarily of the IgG and IgM classes and are capable of fixing complement. However these antibodies do not appear to bind to their corresponding antigen *in vivo* in normal individuals, whereas their presence can be demonstrated in psoriatic scale[84]. This has formed the basis for the following pathogenic pathway proposed by Beutner et al[85]. In a psoriatic individual neutrophils enter the skin in response to trauma or an infection, forming Munro abscesses in the stratum corneum. The neutrophils release proteolytic enzymes which unmask the stratum corneum antigen. The vasodilation accompanying this reaction allows the stratum corneum antibodies to enter the epidermis where they bind to the newly exposed antigen. The resultant complement fixation and production of chemoattractant factors leads to a further influx of neutrophils and exposure of stratum corneum antigen perpetuating the process. Although this hypothesis appears plausible, it does not encompass certain features of this disease, such as its association with arthritis. Furthermore, the increased epidermal growth rate cannot be accounted for convincingly by this hypothesis. It also raises the question as to why Koebnerizing trauma does not lead eventually to psoriasis in normal individuals. The

observation that the stratum corneum antibody is not
present in the early, pre-pinpoint lesion[86] suggests that this
system cannot trigger psoriasis, but does not exclude the
possibility of its involvement in the maintenance of a
psoriatic lesion.

(b) *Anti-basal cell nuclear antibodies.* An antibody predominantly reactive with basal cell nuclei has been demonstrated on the membranes of circulating lymphoid cells
and neutrophils in psoriasis patients[87]. This antibody does
not occur in healthy controls, does not fix complement
and only reacts with nuclei of epidermal cells in uninvolved
skin of psoriatic individuals. These observations have led
Cormane and colleagues[87] to propose a mechanism for the
pathogenesis of psoriasis which involves the interaction of
these antibodies, detached from locally recruited lymphoid
cells and neutrophils, with antigenic receptors on the membranes of basal cells inducing a shift of cells from the
resting phase into the proliferating pool. However, these
antibodies could have a regulatory rather than stimulatory
effect on proliferation[78].

2. Cellular Components

T lymphocytes, monocytes, neutrophils
T Lymphocytes   As described earlier in the chapter, the eruption of a psoriatic lesion is associated with the influx of T
helper (T_H) cells into the epidermis where they are observed,
in an activated state (HLA-DR +), in close proximity to HLA-
DR + Langerhans cells[12]. Langerhans cells are very efficient
antigen-presenting cells which will present antigen, in conjunction with HLA-DR antigen, to T_H cells. Conversely, in the
resolving lesion an increased epidermal entry and activation of
T suppressor (T_S) cells is observed[12]. These findings argue
strongly for an on-going specific immune response in the psoriatic lesion. The presentation of antigen by an antigen-presenting cell to antigen-specific T_H cells results in activation of

the latter and the subsequent release of substances that stimulate many different cell types, including keratinocytes[85]. This has formed the basis for a hypothesis by Valdimarsson and colleagues[89] which proposes that a factor (epidermal proliferation factor, EPF) released by activated T_H cells within the epidermal compartment of a psoriatic lesion is responsible for the stimulation of epidermal growth. Stimulation of epidermal growth would, in turn, result in enhanced production of epidermal thymocyte-activating factor (ETAF) by keratinocytes. ETAF is chemotactic for T lymphocytes[90] and may therefore help to attract these cells from the dermis into the epidermis. It also activates thymic lymphocytes and is similar if not identical to interleukin-1[91]. Thus increased production of ETAF may, in turn, stimulate T_H cells to generate more EPF, resulting in a vicious circle that could be responsible for the persistence and enlargement of psoriatic lesions (Figure 3.3).

Not only the spontaneous resolution of psoriatic lesions, but also the Koebner phenomenon and several histological and biochemical features of active and chronic lesions can be understood in the context of this hypothesis, i.e. that psoriasis is a T cell-mediated disease. In support of this notion are the findings of a recent study[92] which showed that lesional psoriatic epidermal cells are more active in stimulating autologous T cell proliferation than cells from uninvolved psoriatic or normal epidermis. In addition supernatants from antigen-stimulated peripheral blood mononuclear cells from psoriatic patients have less inhibitory and more enhancing effect on Hela cell proliferation than supernatants from normal subjects[93].

The nature of the putative antigen in psoriasis is unknown, but candidates include bacterial, viral and autoantigens (see Aetiology of psoriasis). Virus-like particles have been demonstrated in psoriatic lesions[94]. Furthermore, the cross-reactivity of monoclonal antibodies against streptococcal antigens to the epidermal compartment of skin suggest that a streptococcal infection could lead to an autoimmune reaction against self-antigens[95]. Valdimarsson et al.[89] postulate that psoriasis is associated with abnormal accumulation of T cell-activating antigens in the dermis; causes could involve different interacting combinations of several genetic and environmental factors including HLA and complement-dependent mechanisms for presentation and elimination of antigens. Indeed, there are numerous reports describing defects of cell-mediated immunity in psoriasis. *In vivo* these include a depressed responsiveness to sensitization with chemicals that induce an allergic contact dermatitis, which corrects with therapy[96], and decreased delayed reactivity to intradermal challenge with antigen[97].

In vitro, the proliferative response by psoriatic lymphocytes to mitogens has been reported to be depressed. Whilst one group showed that the greater the extent of skin lesions, the lower the response to phytohaemagglutinin (PHA)[98], another found lymphocyte transformation with PHA to be relatively normal in psoriatic patients but noted a marked decrease in lymphocyte response to Concanavalin-A (Con-A)[99]. Fur-

---

Defects of cell-mediated immunity in psoriasis
- Depressed response to contact allergen
- Decreased delayed response to intradermal challenge with antigen
- Depressed response to mitogens
- Impaired γ-IFN production on Con-A stimulation
- Normal and decreased numbers of T lymphocytes

a)

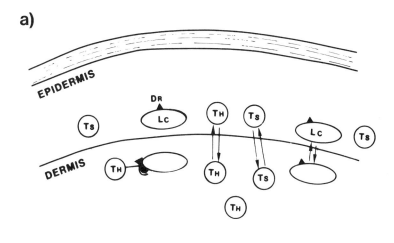

b)

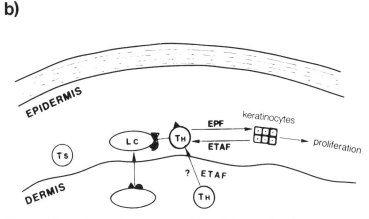

Figure 3.3 Schematic representation of the mechanisms proposed to initiate psoriatic lesions: **(a)** uninvolved; and **(b)** early lesional skin. TH = Helper T cells; TS = suppressor T cells; Lc = Langerhans cells; ▲ = HLA-DR molecules; ● = putative psoriasis antigen(s); EPF = epidermal proliferation factor; ETAF = epidermal T-cell activating factor

thermore, Goan and colleagues[100] recently showed that peripheral blood mononuclear cells from psoriatic patients showed impaired γ-interferon (γ-IFN) production upon Con-A, but not PHA or pokeweed mitogen, stimulation suggesting that psoriatic lymphocytes are unable to respond to weak mitogenic stimuli. It was proposed that the disproportionate depression of Con-A versus normal PHA reactivity might indicate a deficiency of T suppressor cells; this could explain the occurrence of autoantibodies, immune complexes and elevated levels of immunoglobulins in psoriasis[99]. However, conflicting results for T suppressor, and indeed total and helper T cell numbers in peripheral blood of patients with psoriasis have been reported. Any reduction is probably secondary to the extent of lesions[11].

Thus patients with psoriasis appear to have an altered cell-mediated immune status of unknown cause which is not secondary to abnormal numbers of T lymphocytes or subclasses of T lymphocytes.

Monocytes   Abnormalities of monocyte function in psoriasis include increased chemotaxis to various agents, which persists in disease-free individuals and does not correlate with extent of disease[101], increased reduction of nitroblue tetrazolium (NBT)[101], and significantly higher phagocytic and bacteriocidal capacity relative to monocytes from normal subjects[102]. When monocytes ingest opsonized zymosan particles the activation of the hexose monophosphate shunt gives rise to unstable oxygen intermediates that can be monitored as chemiluminescence; monocytes from psoriasis patients peak sooner than normal[103].

Recently, Volk et al.[104] demonstrated that a decreased proportion of peripheral blood monocytes from psoriatic patients expressed HLA-DR antigens compared to normal; this may

---

Abnormalities of monocyte function
- Increased chemotaxis
- Increased reduction of NBT
- Increased phagocytic and bacteriocidal activity
- Increased chemiluminescence on ingestion of zymosan

affect their antigen-presenting function. Furthermore the sera of psoriatic patients contained one or more factors that interfered with the γ-IFN-mediated induction of HLA-DR antigen expression on cultured monocytes of the same patients[104]. These findings may be of relevance to the proposal that psoriatic individuals are unable to eliminate T cell-activating antigens which, as a result, accumulate in the skin.

Neutrophils With one exception neutrophil proliferation, maturation and deployment seem to be unaffected in psoriasis. That exception is the observation that peripheral blood neutrophil counts are elevated in untreated patients with psoriasis even in the absence of infection[105]. However, although statistically significant for psoriatic patients as a whole, this increase is often not out of the normal range for individual patients. The movement of neutrophils into tissue requires firstly their attachment to endothelial walls. An *in vitro* adherence assay designed to measure this function showed that neutrophils from psoriatic patients had increased adherence[105], and the amount of adherence correlated with disease severity. Several chemotactic factors have been identified in psoriatic lesions which could be responsible for the influx of neutrophils into the epidermis, such as complement fragments, 12-HETE and LTB_4, as discussed earlier. Studies of neutrophil chemotaxis *in vitro* have produced conflicting results. However, it does appear that neutrophils in patients with psoriasis are altered in their capacity for chemotaxis, that such alterations are mediated by serum factors and that they tend to be in the direction of increased activity.

The observation that lithium carbonate will exacerbate psoriasis[106] has lent support to the notion that neutrophils play a prominent role in the pathogenesis of psoriasis. However, its mechanism of action is unclear; as well as affecting neutrophil function, lithium inhibits adenyl cyclase and alters immune function, as discussed earlier.

Thus the function of neutrophils may be distorted in psoriasis, but these alterations do not appear to be intrinsic to the neutrophil itself, but induced by its environment. The role of neutrophils in the psoriatic process is unlikely, therefore, to be of a primary nature.

CONCLUSIONS

Although there are abnormalities in various biochemical pathways, and functions of several cell types are altered in psoriasis, most of these defects do not appear to be of a primary nature. The possible exceptions to this are defects of the cell-mediated immune system, which may result in accumulation of antigens in the skin, and of psoriatic keratinocytes which as a consequence proliferate abnormally. These two defects are not mutually exclusive; on the contrary they are very compatible. The pathogenic process appears to be mediated by T lymphocytes; in addition humoral factors are required for expression or non-expression of disease.

REFERENCES

1. Lever, W. F. and Schaumberg-Lever, G. (1983). Psoriasis. In *Histopathology of the Skin*, pp. 139–146. (Philadelphia: Lippincott)
2. Ryan, T. J. (1980). Microcirculation in psoriasis: blood vessels, lymphatics and tissue fluid. *Pharmacol. Ther.*, **10**, 27–64
3. Pinkus, H. and Mehregan, A. H. (1966). The primary histologic lesion of seborrheic dermatitis and psoriasis. *J. Invest. Dermatol.*, **46**, 109–116
4. Braverman, I. M. and Sibley, J. (1982). Role of the microcirculation in the treatment and pathogenesis of psoriasis. *J. Invest. Dermatol.*, **78**, 12–17
5. Klemp, P. and Staberg, B. (1983). Cutaneous blood flow in psoriasis. *J. Invest. Dermatol.*, **81**, 503–506
6. Weinstein, G. D. (1971). Biochemical and pathophysiological rationale for methotrexate in psoriasis. *Ann. N. Y. Acad. Sci.*, **186**, 452–466
7. Mansbridge, J. N., Knapp, A. M. and Strefling, A. M. (1984). Evidence for an alternative pathway of keratinocyte maturation in psoriasis from an antigen found in psoriatic but not normal epidermis. *J. Invest. Dermatol.*, **83**, 296–301
8. Stingl, G., Wolff, K., Diem, E., Baumgartner, G. and Knapp, W. (1977). In situ identification of lymphoreticular cells in benign and

malignant infiltrates by membrane receptor sites. *J. Invest. Dermatol.*, **69**, 231–235

9. Bjerke, J. E., Krogh, H. K. and Matre, R. (1978). Characterisation of mononuclear cell infiltrate in psoriatic lesions. *J. Invest. Dermatol.*, **71**, 340–343

10. Bos, J. D., Hulsebosch, H. J., Krieg, S. R., Bakker, P. M. and Cormane, R. H. (1983). Immunocompetent cells in psoriasis: in situ immuno-phenotyping by monoclonal antibodies. *Arch. Dermatol. Res.*, **275**, 181–189

11. Baker, B. S. Swain, A. F., Valdimarsson, H. and Fry, L. (1984a). T-cell subpopulations in the blood and skin of patients with psoriasis. *Br. J. Dermatol.*, **110**, 37–44

12. Baker, B. S., Swain, A. F., Fry, L. and Valdimarsson, H. (1984b). Epidermal T lymphocytes and HLA-DR expression in psoriasis. *Br. J. Dermatol.*, **110**, 555–564

13. Kohler, G. and Milstein, C. (1975). Continuous cultures of fused cells secreting antibody to predefined specificity. *Nature*, **256**, 495–497

14. Baker, B. S., Swain, A. F., Griffiths, C. E. M., Leonard, J. N., Fry, L. and Valdimarsson, H. (1985). Epidermal T lymphocytes and dendritic cells in chronic plaque psoriasis: the effects of PUVA treatment. *Clin. Exp. Immunol.*, **61**, 526–534

15. Norholm-Pederson, A. (1952). Infections and psoriasis. *Acta Dermato-Venerol.*, **32**, 159–167

16. Whyte, H. J. and Baughman, R. D. (1964). Acute guttate psoriasis and streptococcal infection. *Arch. Dermatol.*, **89**, 350–356

17. Seville, R. H. (1979). Stress and psoriasis. *Br. J. Dermatol.*, **100**, 614–616

18. Marks, R. (1978). Epidermal activity in the involved and uninvolved skin of patients with psoriasis. *Br. J. Dermatol.*, **98**, 399–404

19. Russell, D. H., Combest, W. L., Durell, E. A., Stawiski, M. A., Anderson, T. F. and Vorhees, J. J. (1978). Glucocorticoid inhibits elevated polyamine biosynthesis in psoriasis. *J. Invest. Dermatol.*, **71**, 177–181

20. Fraki, J. E., Briggaman, R. A. and Lazarus, G. S. (1983). Transplantation of psoriatic skin onto nude mice. *J. Invest. Dermatol.*, **80**, 031s–035s

21. Plummer, N. A., Hensby, C. N., Warin, A. P., Camp, R. D. and Greaves, M. W. (1978). Prostaglandin E_2, $F_{2\alpha}$ and arachidonic acid levels in irradiated and unirradiated skin of psoriatic patients receiving PUVA treatment. *Clin. Exp. Dermatol.*, **3**, 367–369

22. Wiley, H. E. and Weinstein, G. D. (1979). Abnormal proliferation in involved psoriatic epidermis: differential induction by saline, propranolol and tape stripping *in vivo*. *J. Invest. Dermatol.*, **73**, 545–547

23. Krueger, G. G., Chambers, D. A. and Shelby, J. (1981). Involved and uninvolved skin from psoriatic subjects: are they equally diseased? *J. Clin. Invest.*, **68**, 1548–1557

24. Haftek, M., Ortonne, J.-P., Staquet, M.-J., Viac, J. and Thivolet, J. (1981). Normal and psoriatic human skin grafts on 'nude' mice:

morphological and immunochemical studies. *J. Invest. Dermatol.*, **76**, 48–52

25. Skerrow, D. and Hunter, I. (1978). Protein modifications during the keratinisation of normal and psoriatic human epidermis. *Biochim. Biophys. Acta*, **537**, 474–484

26. Mali, J. W. H. (1979). Psoriasis: a dynamic disease. *Br. J. Dermatol.*, **101**, 725–730

27. Gommans, J. M., Bergers, M., Van Erp, P. E. J., Van Den Hurk, J. M. A., Mier, P. D. and Roelfzema, H. (1979). Studies on the plasma membrane of normal and psoriatic keratinocytes. I. Preparation of material and morphological characterisation. *Br. J. Dermatol.*, **101**, 407–413

28. King, C. S., Nicholls, S., Barton, S. and Marks, R. (1979). Is the stratum corneum of uninvolved skin abnormal? *Acta Dermato-Venereol.* (Suppl. 59), **85**, 95–100

29. Rust, S., Harth, P. and Herrmann, F. (1970). Untersuchungen der freien Fettsauren im Hautoberflachenfett von Psoriatikern. *Arch. Klin. Exp. Dermatol.*, **238**, 207–211

30. Gara, A., Estrada, E., Rothman, S. and Lorincz, A. L. (1964). Deficient cholesterol esterifying ability of lesion-free skin surface in psoriatic individuals. *J. Invest. Dermatol.*, **43**, 559–564

31. Aiba, S. and Tagami, H. (1984). HLA-DR expression on the keratinocyte surface in dermatoses characterised by lymphocyte exocytosis (eg. pityriasis rosea). *Br. J. Dermatol.*, **111**, 285–294

32. Basham, T. Y., Nickoloff, B. J., Merigan, T. C. and Morhenn, V. B. (1984). Recombinant gamma interferon induces HLA-DR expression on cultured human keratinocytes. *J. Invest. Dermatol.*, **83**, 88–90

33. Nickoloff, B. J., Basham, T. Y., Merigan, T. C. and Morhenn, V. B. (1984). Antiproliferative effects of recombinant α- and γ-interferons on cultured human keratinocytes. *Lab. Invest.*, **51**, 697–701

34. Kariniemi, A.-L. (1977). Effect of human leucocyte interferon on DNA synthesis in human psoriatic skin cultured in diffusion chambers. *Acta Pathol. Microbiol. Scand. Sect. A*, **85**, 270–272

35. Schulze, H.-J. and Mahrle, G. (1986). Effect of interferons (r IFN-alpha 2, r IFN-gamma) on DNA synthesis and HLA-DR expression in psoriasis. *Arch. Dermatol. Res.*, **278**, 416–418

36. Briggaman, R. A. and Wheeler, C. E. Jr (1980). Nude mouse–human skin graft model. III. Studies on generalised psoriasis. *J. Invest. Dermatol.*, **74**, 262

37. Baden, H. P., Kubilus, J. and MacDonald, M. J. (1981). Normal and psoriatic keratinocytes and fibroblasts compared in culture. *J. Invest. Dermatol.*, **76**, 53–55

38. Saiag, P., Coulomb, B., Lebreton, C., Bell, E. and Dubertret, L. (1985). Psoriatic fibroblasts induce hyperproliferation of normal keratinocytes in a skin equivalent model in vitro. *Science*, **230**, 669–672

39. Braun-Falco, O. and Christophers, E. (1974). Structural aspects of initial psoriatic lesions. *Arch. Dermatol. Forsch.*, **251**, 95–110

40. Kulka, J. P. (1964). Microcirculatory impairments as a factor in

inflammatory tissue damage. *Ann. N.Y. Acad. Sci.*, **116**, 1018–1044

41. Braverman, I. M. and Sibley, J. (1982). Role of the microcirculation in the treatment and pathogenesis of psoriasis. *J. Invest. Dermatol.*, **78**, 12–17

42. Braverman, I. M. and Yen, A. (1977). Ultrastructural study of the human dermal microcirculation. II. The capillary loops of the dermal papillae. *J. Invest. Dermatol.*, **68**, 44–52

43. Vorhees, J. J. and Duell, E. A. (1971). Psoriasis as a possible defect of the adenyl cyclase-cyclic AMP cascade: a defective chalone mechanism. *Arch. Dermatol.*, **104**, 352–358

44. Aso, K., Orenberg, E. K. and Farber, E. M. (1975). Reduced epidermal cyclic AMP accumulation following prostaglandin stimulation: Its possible role in the pathophysiology of psoriasis. *J. Invest. Dermatol.*, **65**, 375–378

45. Gommans, J. M., Bergers, M., Van Erp, P. E. J., Van Den Hurk, J. J., Van De Kerkhof, P., Mier, P. F. and Roelfzema, H. (1979). Studies on the plasma membrane of normal and psoriatic keratinocytes. *Br. J. Dermatol.*, **101**, 413–419

46. Iizuka, H., Adachi, K., Halprin, K. M. and Levine, V. (1978). Cyclic nucleotide-phosphodiesterase in the uninvolved and involved skin of psoriasis. *J. Invest. Dermatol.*, **70**, 246–249

47. Vorhees, J. J. (1982). Psoriasis as a possible defect of the adenyl cyclase-cyclic AMP cascade. *Arch. Dermatol.*, **118**, 862–868

48. Fernandez, L. A. and Fox, R. A. (1980). Perturbation of the human immune system by lithium. *Clin. Exp. Immunol.*, **41**, 527–532

49. Arntzen, N., Kavli, G. and Volden, G. (1984). Psoriasis provoked by beta blocking agents. *Acta Dermato-Venereal. (Stockh.)*, **64**, 346–348

50. Rusin, L. J., Duell, E. A. and Vorhees, J. J. (1978). Papaverine and Ro20–1724 inhibit cyclic nucleotide phosphodiesterase activity and increase cyclic AMP levels in psoriatic epidermis in vitro. *J. Invest. Dermatol.*, **71**, 154–156

51. Anderson, R., Gatner, E., Imkamp, F. and Kok, S. H. (1980). In vivo effects of propranolol on some cellular and humoral immune functions in a group of patients with lepromatous leprosy. *Lepr. Rev.*, **51**, 137–148

52. Marcelo, C. L., Duell, E. A., Stawiski, M. A., Anderson, T. F. and Vorhees, J. J. (1979). Cyclic nucleotide levels in psoriatic and normal keratomed epidermis. *J. Invest. Dermatol.*, **72**, 20–24

53. Adachi, K., Aoyagi, T., Nemoto, O., Halprin, K. M. and Levine, V. (1981). Epidermal cyclic GMP is increased in psoriatic lesions. *J. Invest. Dermatol.*, **76**, 19–20

54. Proctor, M. S., Wilkinson, D. I., Orenberg, E. K. and Farber, E. M. (1979). Lowered cutaneous and urinary levels of polyamines with clinical improvement in treated psoriasis. *Arch. Dermatol.*, **115**, 945–949

55. Proctor, M. S., Fletcher, H. V. Jr, Shukla, J. B. and Rennert, O. M. (1975). Elevated spermidine and spermine levels in the blood of psoriasis patients. *J. Invest. Dermatol.*, **65**, 409–411

56. Hammerstrom, S., Hamberg, M., Samuelsson, B., Duell, E. A., Stawiski, M. and Vorhees, J. J. (1975). Increased concentrations of free arachidonic acid, prostaglandins E_2 and $F_{2\alpha}$ and 12L-hydroxy-5,8,10,14-eicosatetraenoic acid (HETE) in epidermis of psoriasis: evidence of perturbed regulation of arachidonic acid levels in psoriasis. *Proc. Natl. Acad. Sci. USA*, **72**, 5130–5134

57. Forster, S., Ilderton, E., Summerly, R. and Yardley, H. J. (1983). The level of phospholipase A_2 activity is raised in the uninvolved epidermis of psoriasis. *Br. J. Dermatol.*, **108**, 103–105

58. Camp, R. D., Mallet, A., Woollard, P., Brain, S., Black, A. K. and Greaves, M. W. (1983). Monohydroxy metabolites of arachidonic and linoleic acids in psoriatic skin. *J. Invest. Dermatol.*, **80**, 359–360

59. Penneys, N. S., Ziboh, V., Lord, J. and Simon, P. (1975). Inhibitor(s) of prostaglandin synthesis in psoriatic plaque. *Nature*, **254**, 351–352

60. Kragballe, K., Desjarlais, L. and Vorhees, J. J. (1985). Leukotrienes B_4, C_4 and D_4 stimulate DNA synthesis in cultured human epidermal keratinocytes. *Br. J. Dermatol.*, **113**, 43–52

61. Lewis, R. A. and Austen, K. F. (1981). Mediation of local homeostasis and inflammation by leukotrienes and other mast cell-dependent components. *Nature*, **293**, 103–108

62. Ellis, C. N., Fallon, J. D., Heezen, J. L. and Vorhees, J. J. (1983). Topical indomethacin exacerbates lesions of psoriasis. *J. Invest. Dermatol.*, **80**, 362

63. Kragballe, K. and Herlin, T. (1983) Benoxaprofen improves psoriasis: a double-blind study. *Arch. Dermatol.*, **119**, 548–552

64. Bray, M. A. (1980). Prostaglandins: fine tuning the immune system? *Immunol. Today*, **2**, 65–69

65. Cantieri, J. S., Graff, G. and Goldberg, N. D. (1980). Cyclic GMP metabolism in psoriasis: activation of soluble epidermal guanylate cyclase by arachidonic acid and 12-hydroxy-5,8,10,14-eicosatetraenoic acid. *J. Invest. Dermatol.*, **74**, 234–237

66. Fraki, J. E., Briggaman, R. A. and Lazarus, G. S. (1983). Transplantation of psoriatic skin onto nude mice. *J. Invest. Dermatol.*, **80**, 031s–035s

67. Lazarus, G. S., Yost, F. J. and Thomas, C. A. (1977). Polymorphonuclear leukocytes: Possible mechanism of accumulation in psoriasis. *Science.*, **198**, 1162–1163

68. Fraki, J. E., Lazarus, G. S., Gilgor, R. S., Marchase, P. and Singer, K. H. (1983). Correlation of epidermal plasminogen activator activity with disease activity in psoriasis. *Br. J. Dermatol.*, **108**, 39–44

69. Vickers, H. R. and Sneddon, I. B. (1963). Psoriasis and hypoparathyroidism. *Br. J. Dermatol.*, **75**, 419–421

70. Van der Kerkhof, P. C. M. and Van Erp, P. E. J. (1983). Calmodulin levels are grossly elevated in the psoriatic lesion. *Br. J. Dermatol.*, **108**, 217–218

71. Tucker, W. F. C., MacNeil, S., Bleehen, S. S. and Tomlinson, S. (1984). Biologically active calmodulin levels are elevated in both involved and uninvolved epidermis in psoriasis. *J. Invest. Dermatol.*, **82**, 298–299

72. Eyre, R. W. and Krueger, G. G. (1982). Interrelations of skin involved and uninvolved with psoriasis to injury and disease activity: Koebner and reverse Koebner reactions. *Br. J. Dermatol.*, **106**, 153–159

73. Stankler, L. (1969). Blood and tissue factors influencing the Koebner reaction in psoriasis. *Br. J. Dermatol.*, **81**, 207–212

74. Heiskell, C. L., Reed, W. B., Weimer, H. E., Becker, S. W. and Carpenter, C. M. (1962). Serum profiles in psoriasis and arthritis. *Arch. Dermatol.*, **85**, 64–71

75. Hall, R. P., Peck, G. and Lawley, J. T. (1981). Detection of IgA immune complexes in patients with psoriasis. *Clin. Res.*, **29**, 597A

76. Guilhou, J.-J., Clot, J., Meynadier, J. and Lapinski, H. (1976) Immunological aspects of psoriasis. I. Immunoglobulins and anti-IgG factors. *Br. J. Dermatol.*, **94**, 501–507

77. Glinski, W., Obalek, S., Langner, A., Jablonska, S. and Haftek, M. (1978). Defective function of T lymphocytes in psoriasis. *J. Invest. Dermatol.*, **70**, 105–110

78. Krueger, G. G. (1981). Psoriasis: current concepts of its etiology and pathogenesis. In: Dobson, R. L. and Thiers, B. H. (eds), *1981 Year Book of Dermatology*, pp.13–70. (Chicago: Year Book Publishing Company).

79. Krueger, G. G., Eyre, R. W., Torres, A. R. and Chambers, D. A. (1981). The Koebner and reverse Koebner reaction in psoriasis; interrelations and correlations with serum factor. *Clin. Res.*, **29**, 603A

80. Krueger, G. G., Chambers, D. A., Stubbs, J. D., Jederberg, W. W. and Torres, A. R. (1982). A role for humoral factors in psoriasis. *J. Lab. Clin. Med.*, **99**, 275–287

81. Wahba, A., Cohen, H., Bar-Eli, M. and Callily, R. (1979). Neutrophil chemotaxis in psoriasis. *Acta Dermato-Venereol.*, **59**, 441–445

82. Majewski, S., Tigalonowa, M., Jablonska, S., Polakowski, I. and Janczura, E. (1987). Serum samples from patients with active psoriasis enhance lymphocyte-induced angiogenesis and modulate endothelial cell proliferation. *Arch. Dermatol.*, **123**, 221–225

83. Krogh, H. K., Maeland, A. J. and Tonder, O. (1972). Indirect haemagglutination for demonstration of antibodies to stratum corneum of skin. *Int. Arch. Allergy*, **42**, 493–502

84. Krogh, H. K. and Tonder, O. (1973). Antibodies in psoriatic scales. *Scand. J. Immunol.*, **2**, 45–51

85. Beutner, E. H., Binder, W. L., Jablonska, S. and Kumar, V. (1982). Immunofluorescence findings on stratum corneum antibodies, antigens and their reaction in vitro and in vivo as related to repair and psoriasis. In: Beutner, E. H. (ed.), *Autoimmunity in Psoriasis*, pp. 53–80. (Boca Raton, FL: CRC Press)

86. Jablonska, S., Beutner, E. H., Chorzelski, T. P., Jarzabek-Chorzelska, M., Rzesa, G., Chowaniec, O. and Maciejowska, E. (1982). IF studies of psoriatic scales and induced psoriatic lesions (Koebner phenomenon). In: Beutner, E. H. (ed.), *Autoimmunity in Psoriasis*, pp. 95–110. (Boca Raton, FL: CRC Press)

87. Cormane, R. H., Hunyadi, J. and Hamerlinck, F. (1976). The role of

lymphoid cells and polymorphonuclear leukocytes in the pathogenesis of psoriasis. *J. Dermatol.*, **3**, 247–259

88. Korszun, A.-K., Wilton, J. M. and Johnson, N. W. (1981). The *in vivo* effects of lymphokines on mitotic activity and keratinisation in guinea pig epidermis. *J. Invest. Dermatol.*, **76**, 433–437

89. Valdimarsson, H., Baker, B. S., Jonsdottir, I. and Fry, L. (1986). Psoriasis: a disease of abnormal keratinocyte proliferation induced by T lymphocytes. *Immunol. Today*, **7**, 256–259

90. Sauder, D. N. (1984). Epidermal cytokines: properties of epidermal cell thymocyte activating factor (ETAF). *Lymph. Res.*, **3**, 145–151

91. Luger, T. A., Stadler, B. M., Katz, S. I. and Oppenheim, J. (1981). Epidermal cell (keratinocyte)-derived thymocyte-activating factor (ETAF). *J. Immunol.*, **127**, 1493–1498

92. Schopf, R. E., Hoffman, A., Jung, M., Morsches, B. and Bork, K. (1986). Stimulation of T cells by autologous mononuclear leukocytes and epidermal cells in psoriasis. *Arch. Dermatol. Res.*, **279**, 89–94

93. Krueger, G. G. and Jederberg, W. W. (1980). Alteration of Hela cell growth equilibrium by supernatants of peripheral blood mononuclear cells from normal and psoriatic subjects. *J. Invest. Dermatol.*, **74**, 148–153

94. Bjerke, J. R. Haukenes, G., Livden, J. K., Matre, R. and Degre, M. (1983). Activated T lymphs, interferon and retrovirus-like particles in psoriatic lesions. *Arch. Dermatol.*, **119**, 955–956

95. Swerlick, R. A., Cunningham, M. W. and Hall, N. K. (1986). Monoclonal antibodies cross-reactive with Group A streptococci and normal and psoriatic human skin. *J. Invest. Dermatol.*, **87**, 367–371

96. Obalek, S., Haftek, M. and Glinski, W. (1977). Immunological studies in psoriasis. *Dermatologica.*, **155**, 13–23

97. Krueger, G. G., Hill, H. R. and Jederberg, W. W. (1978). Inflammatory and immune cell function in psoriasis – a subtle disorder. I. In vivo and in vitro survey. *J. Invest. Dermatol.*, **71**, 189–194

98. Levantine, A. and Brostoff, J. (1975). Immunological responses of patients with psoriasis and the effect of treatment with methotrexate. *Br. J. Dermatol.*, **93**, 659–668

99. Guilhou, J.-J., Clot, J. and Meynadier, J. (1977). T cell defect in Psoriasis: Further studies on membrane markers and T cell functions from 60 patients. *Arch. Dermatol. Res.*, **260**, 163–166

100. Goan, S.-R., Volk, H. D., Eichhorn, I. and Diezel, W. (1986). Differences in interferon-gamma response of psoriatic lymphocytes to stimulation with various mitogens. *Biomed. Biochim. Acta*, **45**, 903–906

101. Krueger, G. G., Jederberg, W. W., Ogden, B. E. and Reese, D. L. (1978). Inflammatory and immune cell function in psoriasis. II. Monocyte function, lymphokine production. *J. Invest. Dermatol.*, **71**, 195–201

102. Bar-Eli, M., Gallily, R., Cohen, H. A. and Wahba, A. (1979). Monocyte function in psoriasis. *J. Invest. Dermatol.*, **73**, 147–149

103. Krueger, G. G. and Jederberg, W. W. (1981). Mononuclear cell func-

tion and its relative potential in the pathogenesis of psoriasis. In: Beutner, E. H. (ed.), *Psoriasis.* (Cleveland: CRC Press)

104. Volk, H.-D., Diezel, W., Waschke, S. R., Barthelmes, H., Grunow, R., Fiebig, H. and Sonnichsen, N. (1985). Abnorme HLA-DR-Antigen Expression an Monozyten von Patienten mit Lupus erythematodes viszeralis und Psoriasis vulgaris. *Dermatol. Monatsschr.,* **171,** 308-311

105. Sedgwick, J. B., Bergstresser, P. R. and Hurd, E. R. (1980). Increased granulocyte adherence in psoriasis and psoriatic arthritis. *J. Invest. Dermatol.,* **74,** 81-84

106. Skoven, I. and Thormann, J. (1979). Lithium compound treatment and psoriasis. *Arch. Dermatol.,* **115,** 1185-1187

4

ECZEMA: CLINICAL FEATURES

R. J. CLAYTON

Eczema is the name given to a broad clinical variety of inflammatory skin diseases. To the uninitiated the spectrum of clinical features can be confusing. For example, eczema can present merely as redness or oedema, mimicking urticaria or angio-oedema. Other cases show a profusion of signs with blistering, weeping and crusting, or thickened pigmented areas of skin with scaling. Scratch marks are frequently a feature.

Some dermatologists use dermatitis and eczema synonymously. It would seem preferable not to use the term dermatitis, which means, vaguely, inflammation of the skin, and therefore could apply to other non-eczematous inflammatory disorders. Also dermatitis features in the name of some dermatological conditions, e.g. dermatitis artefacta, dermatitis herpetiformis and exfoliative dermatitis.

Eczema accounts for a large proportion of skin disease. Although some cases may easily be classified, others are not. There may be clinical overlap in the same patient. However, classification is very useful in predicting natural history and therefore response to treatment. The following is a useful, well-accepted guide:

Exogenous (contact) eczema
Irritant – related to direct injury
Allergic – immunologically mediated

Endogenous eczema
Seborrhoeic
  infantile
  adult
Pompholyx (hands and feet)
Nummular or discoid
Hypostatic (varicose)
Atopic

Others
Juvenile plantar dermatosis
Pityriasis alba
Asteatotic eczema
Exfoliative dermatitis, i.e. eczema all over
Photosensitive

All the above have the potential to become secondarily infected, often from scratching. All types of eczema may be either:

(1) Acute with blisters or bullae, and later weeping or crusting. These lesions are very inflamed with erythema and oedema. It occurs especially in contact and hypostatic eczema and pompholyx.
(2) Subacute eczema shows scaling with inflammation and redness and occasional small blisters, e.g. nummular or seborrhoeic eczema.
(3) Chronic, which is merely scaly with minimal inflammation and redness. This is the commonest type and it often becomes lichenified and thickened from scratching and rubbing.

Types of eczema

Exogenous
- Irritant
- Allergic

Endogenous
- Atopic
- Seborrhoeic
- Discoid
- Gravitational
- Hand and foot (pompholyx)
- Asteatotic

SEBORRHOEIC ECZEMA IN ADULTS

Seborrhoeic eczema is a very common skin condition occurring predominantly in men and in the 16–50 age group. It is so called because it occurs predominantly in areas where sebaceous glands are plentiful. There is, however, no relation between the activity of the glands and the eczema. The basic seborrhoeic eczema lesion is a red scaly variably defined area. The scales on the face are often described as being greasy, but a lot of patients complain of dryness of the affected areas.

Dandruff can be regarded as a minimal manifestation of seborrhoeic eczema. Virtually all patients with seborrhoeic eczema elsewhere will have scalp involvement, but not everybody with dandruff will suffer other features of seborrhoeic eczema, although they are predisposed. Scalp scaling may be patchy or generalized. Though inflammation with erythema is usual, it may be absent. Scalp scales may accumulate to form plaques, which are often picked. The scalp rash is often contiguous with similar eczema of adjacent, non-hair-bearing areas, behind the ears, where fissures may develop, and on the upper forehead. Marginal blepharitis with redness and itching of the edges of the eyelids may be a feature. The site of beards and moustaches may show scalp-like seborrhoeic eczema, with or without a sterile folliculitis with pustulation. The characteristic facial lesion affects the so-called butterfly area (Figure 4.1), that is the bridge of the nose, and adjacent medial cheeks and nasolabial folds. The redness here causes marked cosmetic disability. This redness is often more pronounced after moderate alcohol ingestion the evening before. Between the eyebrows and the middle of the forehead is another favourite site. Ear involvement results in otitis externa.

Seborrhoeic eczema occurs less commonly on the trunk. It may occur, particularly in men, in the sternal area between the breasts, where there may be general involvement of the upper trunk, usually with a marked follicular element with papules and pustules of the back. Flexural areas are a further site of involvement in some patients, thus seborrhoeic eczema may produce an intertrigo, a rash of opposed skin surfaces. The axillae, groins, natal cleft, and submammary areas (Figure 4.2) may be variably involved. Fissures may develop, and weeping and sweating may predispose to secondary infection. Scales may not be evident in these areas because of friction. These flexural lesions are commoner in older patients, who may develop an extensive rash within a short period.

Seborrhoeic eczema is very variable in its severity and extent, but there is a tendency to chronicity and recurrence. Emotional factors may aggravate, but ultraviolet light is usually helpful after initial aggravation of the erythema.

Diagnosis   Seborrhoeic eczema is not usually difficult to diagnose. Psoriasis may be a problem on the scalp and in the flexures. On the scalp psoriasis occurs as elsewhere with well-defined plaques and silvery scales. It is not as likely as seborrhoeic eczema to produce involvement of all the scalp. In some patients psoriasis is remarkably flexural, producing intertrigo. The appearance here may not be typical because of loss of characteristic scales, as indeed in seborrhoeic eczema.

Other causes of intertrigo must be considered – candida, ringworm of the groins, erythrasma and contact eczemas. A

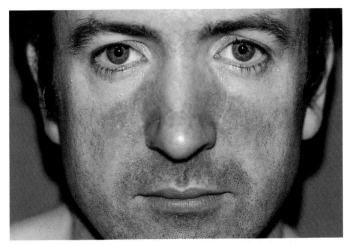

Figure 4.1 Seborrhoeic eczema on the medial cheeks

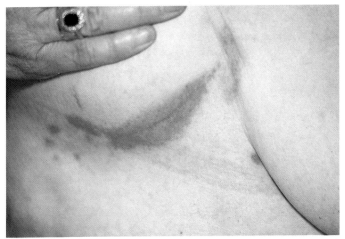

Figure 4.2 Seborrhoeic eczema in the submammary region

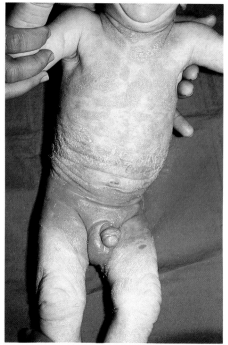

Figure 4.3 Seborrhoeic eczema of infancy; confluent involvement in the napkin area with spread to elsewhere on trunk

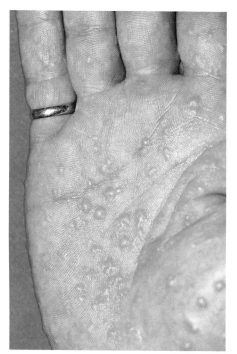

Figure 4.4 Pompholyx eczema; small blisters on the palms

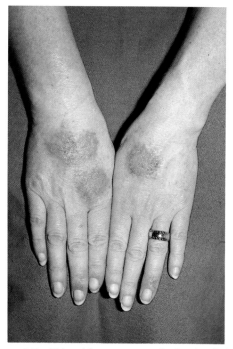

Figure 4.5 Discoid eczema on the back of the hands

rare form of clinically non-blistering pemphigus, foliaceus, may mimic seborrhoeic eczema of the upper trunk.

The 'butterfly' area of the face may also be involved in discoid lupus erythematosus, rosacea and granulomatous conditions, e.g. sarcoidosis.

INFANTILE SEBORRHOEIC ECZEMA

It is convenient clinically to consider this as an eczema, though histologically there are features of psoriasis. It mimics adult seborrhoeic eczema and can occur abruptly, and may quickly become very extensive. Parents are alarmed.

Infantile seborrhoeic eczema starts usually in the first few weeks of life. It is not significantly itchy. There is dramatic well-defined erythema with peripheral scales. Some children who develop 'napkin or ammonia dermatitis' from prolonged contact with urine and/or faeces also have features of seborrhoeic eczema away from the nappy area (Figure 4.3). The seborrhoeic eczema diathesis predisposes to nappy 'dermatitis'. Some patients with seborrhoeic eczema of infancy develop very psoriasiform areas, and some dermatologists prefer to call this napkin psoriasis. Indeed, some patients with infantile seborrhoeic eczema develop psoriasis in later years. Also, some later develop, coincidentally, atopic eczema.

The natural history is generally of a few weeks, even if the condition is not treated. Relapses are most unusual.

POMPHOLYX

The term dyshidrotic eczema for this condition must be disregarded, for it is unrelated to sweating. Pompholyx occurs on the hands and feet, predominantly the palms and soles. Females are affected more often than males, and most cases occur before the age of 40 years. Its appearance and behaviour is thought to be related to the anatomical site. All of the clinical spectrum of eczema is seen. Patients may present acutely with blisters (Figure 4.4), which coalesce, producing itchy bullae. There is minimal erythema. Blisters break down with weeping, and inflammatory oedema. There may be difficulty in moving the fingers to form a fist, and the incapacity of the hand in this situation, and difficulty in walking when the feet are affected, is appreciable in severe cases. An attack resolves spontaneously with eventually more chronic, dry, scaly eczema, within a few weeks. Recurrences are common within weeks or after many years. In a mild case small blisters on the sides of the fingers may be the only physical sign. Asymmetry is unusual. Secondary infection with pustules or ascending lymphangitis is not uncommon.

Other patients present with slower onset of more chronic eczema. Blisters are infrequent. Dry, scaly, lichenified eczema, with dull erythema and fissures of the palms and finger flexures, predominate. This type may extend to the adjacent backs of the hands and onto the lateral dorsae of the feet. Chronic scratching and rubbing may contribute to lichenification. This chronic type may be prolonged between acute attacks. Irritant contact factors at work or in the home will help potentiate it. An acute pompholyx may follow a few weeks after an emotionally traumatic episode. Some patients are coincidentally atopic.

Diagnosis　Nothing mimics acute pompholyx. The diagnosis on the feet is from ringworm, which is often unilateral and may occur with minimal erythema. Skin scrapings should be taken from blister roofs and/or scales. Some patients with inflammatory ringworm on the soles and between the toes develop a non-fungal blistering pompholyx-like reaction of the palms. This is the so-called 'Id' reaction, which is both curious and rare.

Asymmetry will also suggest contact eczema, irritant or allergic, though this is more common on the dorsae and sides of the feet and of the fingers, backs and sides of hands, and fronts of the wrists.

NUMMULAR OR DISCOID ECZEMA

This type of eczema is characterized by coin-shaped areas of moderately well-defined acute, subacute or chronic eczema. They are a few centimetres across. It predominantly occurs in the middle-aged and elderly. The acute lesions show small blisters on an erythematous and oedematous base. Blisters break down leaving small yellow crusts which are not usually secondarily infected. In patients with more extensive disease the lesions are more chronic, with scaly patches and variable lichenification. Only one lesion may be present, usually on the lower leg, but more are usual, developing over weeks or months. The back of the hand (Figure 4.5) is a common site both in men and women. Other favourite areas are the extensor forearms, and in elderly men particularly the lower legs. Trunk lesions occur usually in more extensive disease.

Localized habit scratching or rubbing, especially of the peripheral lesions, may produce marked lichenification, rather than excoriations, mimicking lichen simplex. When there are few lesions scrapings should be taken to exclude ringworm. As in all forms of eczema, contact sensitivity should be considered, but the distribution is rather against this. Nummular eczema lesions come and go over months or a few years, then the condition appears to resolve, but elderly patients are often troubled by more extensive and prolonged disease.

HYPOSTATIC OR VARICOSE ECZEMA

Hypostatic or varicose eczema occurs first on the lower leg or legs, and is associated with varicose veins and other manifestations of stasis. The patient with hypostatic eczema may have, in addition, oedema, purpura, postinflammatory hyperpigmentation and ulceration. Chronic disease is usual. Large overweight women are especially predisposed. The eczema may be acute and blistering or more chronic and scaly. Scaly lesions are often scratched, and linear excoriations may be seen above the ankle. Large blistering areas may weep profusely, necessitating frequent changes of dressings.

Acute flares of eczema may occur spontaneously or following contact sensitivity. Patients with chronic leg ulcers have often had many topical applications applied to their ulcers, and the skin around, and they have a very high incidence of contact problems. The lower legs are the frequent site of trauma, and this may influence the natural history of the eczema and any ulceration.

Acute and chronic cellulitis of the lower leg is frequently seen, especially in large women's legs where there has been prolonged chronic oedema, related to hypostasis. Further swelling and ascending redness with exquisite pain on touching suggest acute cellulitis. The appearances of a chronic cellulitis are often not remarkable. Recurrent episodes of cellulitis and intermittent ulcer infection predispose to scarring about the ankle, and tethering of the skin to subcutaneous elements. A ballooned calf above this results in the so-called inverted champagne bottle, which rather glamorizes an unpleasant condition. These leg problems can obviously significantly affect the mobility of patients, and attention to the hypostasis, as well as the skin problems, is essential.

SECONDARY DISSEMINATION OF ECZEMA

It is convenient at this stage to consider the characteristic feature of eczema to spread away from its primary sites. It is most commonly seen in hypostatic eczema.

In endogenous eczema, spread to distant parts occurs by mechanisms which are little known, but may in part be immunological. In allergic contact eczema the spread is more obvious to further sites of contact. Extension may occur around the areas of primary sites, or may develop at distant sites. About one-third of patients with chronic hypostatic eczema show this phenomenon. The next common group is those with allergic contact eczema, spread occurring both from further contact and endogenous spread. For example, topical neomycin, which has produced contact eczema in a hypostatic area, may produce an eczema on the applying fingers and other odd contact areas, due to increasing contact potential of the neomycin. This is asymmetrical. Most secondary dissemination occurs 'endogenously' following non-specific exacerbation of inflammation at the primary site. This is asymmetrical, and is usually a vesicular eruption with small papules, which later become more chronic, red and scaly. If the primary site remains inflamed, spread of eczema may become very extensive, but with successful treatment of the site the secondary eruption fades.

EXFOLIATIVE DERMATITIS

Secondary dissemination of eczema can occasionally progress to a generalized rash. This is an exfoliative dermatitis. Erythroderma is synonymous. The patient is red and scaly all over. An eczematous exfoliative dermatitis may occur abruptly, within days, or more commonly, over weeks or months, in patients with a long history of moderate to severe eczema. Any type of eczema can progress in this direction. Patients are usually elderly. Younger patients are atopic.

In patients with acute onset of exfoliative dermatitis there may only be the briefest of eczema in the recent past history. Rapidly progressive redness, and later scaling, may be accompanied by fever and malaise. Itching is severe and redness may fluctuate from day to day. The more chronic type appears to follow the relentless progression of a chronic eczema which gets more and more extensive with time. There may be some generalized hair loss with noticeable thinning of the scalp hair; nails may also be lost. There is always enlargement of superficial lymph nodes with chronic disease; this is a non-specific reaction to the generalized rash.

Although in most cases of exfoliative dermatitis there is an underlying eczema, other conditions may be involved; for example psoriasis may become generalized, or there may be a severe drug eruption. Exfoliative dermatitis may also occur secondary to myeloproliferative syndromes, particularly Hodgkin's disease. In these cases histology of the skin shows eczema, but enlarged glands may be malignant. There is also a rare T-cell type of lymphoma, mycosis fungoides, which occurs initially in the skin and may become generalized. In these cases biopsy of eczematous-looking skin shows lymphoma.

There are, of course, cases in which the underlying association of cause is not evident. Some patients with eczematous exfoliative dermatitis have developed lymphoma as long as 2–3 years later. It should be appreciated that exfoliative dermatitis is often a prolonged disease, and associated with a raised metabolic rate, risk of hypothermia – through heat loss through the erythematous skin, increased cardiac output with potential for heart failure, increased percutaneous fluid and protein loss in scales. These hint at the potential problems in the management of these patients.

Atopic Eczema

Atopy is a genetically determined state related to immunological abnormalities. It is characterized by an increase in serum IgE, and therefore susceptibility to familial eczema, asthma, hay fever and anaphylactoid reactions. The aetiology is unknown.

Most patients with atopic eczema in fact have very little eczema. Physical signs are related more to scratching with excoriations, lichenification and secondary infection. There is a family history of atopy in about three-quarters of cases, although the true genetics is obscure. The skin is very dry, and there may be minor degrees of ichthyosis and follicular keratosis pilaris, particularly of the limbs.

The onset of atopic eczema may be at any age after the first month, but between the second and sixth months of life is usual. It is never present at birth. Atopic eczema is the commonest form of juvenile eczema, and itching, often intense, is invariable. Infants or children may rub and scratch for many hours if left to their own devices. Scratching continues during sleep, excoriations leaving blood on the bedclothes.

Infantile atopic eczema may start anywhere, but the face is a common site, followed by the well-described flexural limb eczema of the antecubital fossae (Figure 4.6*), behind the knees, and around the wrists and ankles. The napkin area is not particularly affected. In some infants limb eczema is more extensor than flexor, being over the knees and elbows. This pattern, which occurs in about one-third of patients, may continue into childhood, but other cases become flexor as the child gets older.

The lesions of atopic eczema may be very extensive, with non-specific lymphadenopathy. On the face there can be weeping and crusting, but elsewhere the rash is usually dry unless there is secondary infection. Extensor or flexural lesions are ill-defined and the characteristic exaggerated skin creases of lichenification are obvious. Excoriations are localized, rather than linear, and may surmount oedematous papules. If these are a marked feature clinically, the diagnosis of atopy may be put in doubt. The disease runs a chronic course with remissions and exacerbations, sometimes related to environmental factors and stress. The majority of cases progress into childhood when the flexural element or lichenification are most marked. Typical nummular eczematous areas can occur with vesicles. Pruritis and scratching continues unabated.

A large number of cases of atopic eczema remit in late childhood, though dry skin usually remains. Adult eczema is similar clinically to the childhood type, and generally occurs in those who had particularly troublesome disease. It is unusual, though, after the age of 40.

Patients with atopy are predisposed to localized vasoconstriction which may be evident clinically as a curious pallor of the skin, especially after scratching – white dermographism. They find that sweating often exacerbates symptoms, though

* Facing page 120.

atopy is commoner in temperate climates compared with the tropics.

The skin is particularly susceptible to psychogenic factors, such as worry and anxiety, some of which may result from the eczema itself. Scratching may become very much a habit.

Asthma and hay fever occur in about 40% of patients with eczema. The age of onset of both is later than the eczema. Atopic patients are predisposed to drug hypersensitivity and bites and sting reactions. Any food allergy would appear to be unrelated.

Atopics, because of dryness of their skin, have a reduced resistance to the effects of irritants. Therefore contact factors such as clothing, the weather, working and home environment, as well as frame of mind, influence the natural history.

KAPOSI'S VARICELLIFORM ERUPTION

Atopics, with or without eczema or rash, are predisposed to skin dissemination of herpes simplex virus, and in the past to vaccinia virus – eczema herpeticum, eczema vaccinatum.

About 10 days after herpes simplex there is a rapid onset of generalized umbilicated vesicles, many of which become pustular and weep. New lesions continue to appear for about a week. There is fever with constitutional symptoms and the individual may become very ill. Healing occurs with crusting and scarring. Secondary infection is common. Death may occur from systemic disease, but in most cases it is less extensive with a few dozen vesicular lesions.

OTHER JUVENILE ECZEMAS

Juvenile plantar dermatosis

This is an eczema-like condition occurring on the soles in children and teenagers. It often starts shortly after beginning school. The forefoot proximal to the toes shows scaling and fissuring. Erythema is minimal. The affected skin appears smooth and shiny, and the heels are sometimes involved. Any atopy is thought to be coincidental. This comparatively recently described problem is thought to be related to the wearing of occlusive synthetic-fibre footwear, and friction. Patch testing is unhelpful; though some may be positive, they are not related to the rash. Skin scrapings will exclude fungus.

Pityriasis alba

Although pityriasis alba is common in all races it is most pronounced in the dark-skinned because of associated post-inflammatory hypopigmentation. It occurs predominantly between the age of 4 and 12 years. Its distribution favours the face, with finely scaled hypopigmented areas, mainly on the cheeks. They are a centimetre or two across. White-skinned patients may show mild erythema, but it is not often evident in the very pale-skinned. The second most frequent site is the upper arms; only rarely is it more extensive. The natural history is of many months or a few years. Atopy is thought to be coincidental.

Perioral Eczema

This occurs in lip-licking children who are frequently atopic. The rash is around the mouth and shows lichenified, scaly skin with often painful fissures of the periphery of the lips and adjacent skin. Soreness is a prominent feature, but patients persist in picking off scales. In the very young there may be contributory dribbling or thumb-sucking.

ASTEATOTIC ECZEMA (Eczema craquelé)

This condition occurs in the elderly, particularly on the lower legs. It is characterized by dryness of the skin, with superficial cracking, mimicking a crazy-paving appearance. The cracks may become inflamed and erythematous, but rarely there may be troublesome weeping. It occurs first on the shins, and on surrounding skin, and is unrelated to hypostasis. It develops frequently in hospitalized patients who have more contact with soaps and cleansing agents on the ward than at home. The skin becomes, as it were, degreased. General ill-health and malnutrition contribute, and occasionally cases of myxoedema have presented with this. In an extensive case, most parts of the skin may become affected. These patients may develop irritation and they scratch. Central heating and dryness of the atmosphere contribute to this problem.

CONTACT ECZEMA

Irritant Contact Eczema

Irritant contact eczema is produced by any substance which is capable of producing cell damage in the skin. It depends on the time and frequency of application, the concentration and the state of the individual skin. Most chemicals penetrate the skin to a variable extent. The horny layer may be easily damaged or stripped off, critically altering the capability of the skin to hold water. Homeostatic mechanisms are lost. An agent may produce no reaction when applied once, even for a long time, but repeated exposure will produce chemical change.

An eczematous irritant reaction may follow an accident at work, or in the home, with an acid, alkali or other chemical. There may be a history of single-occasion contact, or a few brief applications. Physical signs appear within 48 hours. The rash occurs at the site or sites of contact, often with a sharp cut-off. Generally, an acute eczema develops with blistering or weeping. Initially there is discomfort and pain with redness and oedema. Severe reactions result in necrosis of the epidermis and potential scarring. Healing occurs spontaneously.

The commonest form of more chronic cumulative damage occurs on the hands and forearms of housewives. It often occurs 2–3 months after the birth of a child, and is related to the alternate wetting and drying with housework and baby care in the presence of soaps and detergents. A variable period of chapping precedes other physical signs. Later a chronic, red, scaly eczematous eruption appears on the backs of the hands, on the sides of the fingers, and the front of the wrists. Later it may become excoriated and lichenified and fissured. The margins are ill-defined. The palms appear to be protected by the thickness there of the keratin layer. Hairdressers who regularly wash hair can get a similar problem.

Other situations where this sort of reaction may occur is in those using engineering cutting oils. Impregnated overalls, or oil getting into the shoes, can enhance the distribution of the rash. As in other eczemas, a severe reaction may, in the predisposed, produce a chronic low-grade eczema, away from sites of contact.

It is not intended here to go into any detail about the various causes of irritant eczemas, for it is a very large subject. This also applies to the next section on contact allergic eczema. The idea is to give a general impression of the clinical problem, and how it may occur[1].

Allergic Contact Eczema

Contact allergy is produced by low molecular weight chemicals by means of a Coombs type IV cellular lymphocytic immunological reaction. Potential allergens, haptens, combine with skin protein after skin contact and become antigenic. Contact allergy is idiosyncratic.

Sensitization may occur 'immediately'; that is after the second contact, the first priming the immune system, or it may occur after a long period of intermittent contact, e.g. chromate used in the building industry. Once acquired contact sensitivity tends to persist for years. Concentration of allergen is irrelevant clinically, for if a patient is sensitized, in theory, only one molecule of the allergen is necessary to initiate the immunological reaction. For example a patient who is primula-sensitive may experience an uncomfortable 'pricking' of the skin the moment he enters a primula-containing room. Multiple sensitivities are common, and cross-sensitization occurs with compounds that are closely related chemically or broken down in the skin to similar components. For example *p*-phenylenediamine present in organic dyes and cosmetics cross-reacts with benzocaine. Sensitization is more likely to occur if a potential allergen is applied to damaged skin, e.g. an eczematous skin. This explains the frequency of sensitivity to various topical medicaments, e.g. neomycin.

Clinical features   The broad spectrum of clinical contact eczema necessitates organized detective work, starting with a detailed history of the complaint, and some knowledge of the patient's habits at work and in the home. Hobbies should be enquired into, and in both men and women, the use of cosmetics.

About two-thirds of all cases of contact allergic eczema affect the hands. Housewives with irritant hand eczema are frequently found to have allergic sensitivity in addition, for example to nickel. The face is another common site, predominantly from medicaments (Figure 4.7), cosmetics and scents. The rash often starts on the eyelids, which may only show oedema, mimicking angio-oedema. Nail varnish and the striking of non-safety matches in front of the face can cause this reaction. Other body areas may show characteristic contact sensitivity patterns, e.g. right around the hair line from hair dyes and applications (no rash on the scalp), a perianal rash, a popular site for the application of medicaments often containing sensitizing local anaesthetics.

The frequency of reactions to certain groups of substances prevents dermatologists from prescribing, e.g. topical antihistamines and local anaesthetics. The chemist sells such appli-

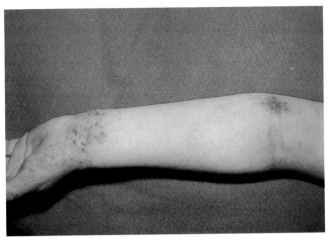

Figure 4.6 Atopic eczema; flexural involvement of the wrist and elbow

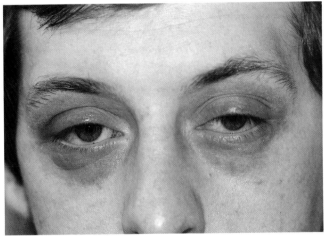

Figure 4.7 Contact eczema on the eyelids from the use of neomycin

cations over the counter, and *MIMS* list many. There is no dermatological indication for any of them, for there are superior alternatives in each case.

Contact allergic sensitivity is a subject in itself, and will doubtless become part of the sub-speciality, industrial dermatitis. The number of potential allergens known is in the thousands, and time and experience is necessary in elucidating the cause of the allergic eczema.

Patch testing Patients thought to have contact allergy are patch tested to an agreed European battery of common allergens. A small amount of each allergen in appropriate concentration, which has been determined by experience, is applied to the skin of the back under occlusion; 48 and 96 hours later the skin is 'read' to determine any sensitivity. An eczematous reaction is positive. Patients tested should be virtually clear of eczema at the time of testing, to prevent false positive reactions which may occur.

It is a good general rule to patch test all patients with hand eczema and eczema of the face. Patients with unusual eczemas, often of bizarre distribution and strikingly unilateral, should also be patch tested. Another situation which should lead to patch testing is the patient who has appeared several times in the clinic with eczema which is unresponsive to treatment. Unexpected positive reactions may be revealed in this way, and possibly a reaction to a topical application previously prescribed.

Table 4.1   Commonly used items containing potential sensitizers

Cement	Creams and ointment bases
Metals	Tars
Nickel	Rosin
Cobalt	Scents and flavours
Rubbers	Dyes
Medicaments	Glues
Lanolin vehicles	
Preservatives in cosmetics	
Plastics	

Table 4.1 is a short list of commonly used items which contain potential sensitizers. They are in no order, and give some idea of the breadth of reactions.

PHOTOSENSITIVE ECZEMA

Photosensitivity which may produce eczema is of two types. The first is produced by chemicals in contact with the skin, which are activated by light exposure. They may be toxic or true allergic reactions. The second is the general photo sensitivity produced following ingestion of a drug, e.g. a thiazide diuretic or tetracycline.

Phototoxic reactions are produced by tars, various plants, dyes and drugs. Clinically, it initially resembles sunburn, with oedema, erythema and bulla formation. Photoallergic reactions are idiosyncratic. They may be produced most commonly by drugs, e.g. phenothiazines, sulphonamides, and ingredients in cosmetic preparations.

Photo patch testing is applied to the elucidation of photo-reactions, and is a specialist procedure.

Some patients with chronic eczema, including atopic, may develop general photosensitivity after some years. The mechanisms involved have not been elucidated.

Reference

1. Cronin, E. (1980). *Contact Dermatitis.* (London: Churchill Livingstone)

5

THE MANAGEMENT OF ECZEMA

J. N. LEONARD

INTRODUCTION

For the majority of patients, eczema is a chronic condition with phases of activity and remission. The active phases can, at best, be controlled by the skilful use of appropriate therapies available to the physician. The learning of these skills will be rewarded by relieving the considerable distress and suffering of affected individuals.

This chapter will first of all consider the therapeutic options that are available, and then place them into a clinical context by discussing their use in the management of different clinical situations.

THERAPEUTIC AGENTS AVAILABLE

Topical Corticosteroids

There can be little argument that topical corticosteroid preparations have revolutionized the management of eczema. They have the combined advantage of being relatively pleasant to use, as compared with the older tar-based alternatives, for example, and they are therapeutically very effective. They have, however, been subject to a great deal of adverse publicity to the extent that, in some cases, the patients' confidence in their safety has been so undermined that they will not consider using them. The source of these criticisms comes from the development of side-effects that came with the over-enthusiastic use of the potent preparations in the early days of clinical usage. The capacity of these agents to produce adverse side-effects is now generally well recognized. It would, in fact, be surprising if such powerful therapeutic agents were free from any risk of ill-effect. There must, however, be a clear distinction made between use and abuse, so that a balanced view of the merits of topical corticosteroids may emerge. Adjunctive non-steroidal therapies, and the tailoring of the strength of the topical corticosteroid application to the severity of the eczema and the sites to be treated, have been successful in reducing the side-effects in all but the most severely affected patients.

Composition of topical corticosteroids

Corticosteroids are crystalline preparations and must be suspended in a suitable vehicle. A proprietary topical corticosteroid preparation has three main constituents: the vehicle, the corticosteroid itself and a preservative.

The vehicle   The vehicle constitutes over 99% (w/v) of a topical corticosteroid preparation. It is thus a major part of the formulation. An ideal vehicle should be easy to apply and remove, be non-toxic, non-irritant and non-allergic. It must also be homogeneous and chemically stable. Topical corticosteroid preparations are, in the main, available as ointments, creams, gels and specialized scalp applications.

(a)   *Ointments* have oil or grease as the continuous phase. They are occlusive, emollient and protective. They resist transepidermal water loss and are therefore hydrating and moisturizing. Ointments can be divided into two main groups – (i) fatty ointments such as Vaseline and

(ii) water-soluble ointments such as polyethylene glycol. Both types are emollient but the former group are more occlusive and have greater hydrating properties. Ointments are most appropriate for dry, flaking, chronic eczemas where their occlusive effect provides a barrier to evaporation of water. Ointments are by their nature sticky, and are not always cosmetically acceptable to the patient.

(b) *Creams* contain oil and water. Oil in water (aqueous) creams are water-miscible, cooling and soothing. They are well absorbed into the skin. They are not occlusive but have a mild moisturizing effect because of their dispersed nature. Water in oil (oily) creams are immiscible in water. They are more occlusive than aqueous creams but less so than ointments. Creams are most appropriately applied to acute weeping eczemas. The corticosteroid is able to mix with the serous exudate, and evaporation of water aids drying.

(c) *Gels* are semi-solid preparations gelled with high molecular weight polymers. They are non-greasy, mix with water, are easy to apply and easy to wash off. They are especially suitable for hairy areas such as the scalp.

(d) *Scalp preparations* are available either as water-based lotions or they are alcohol-based. They are liquid and easy to apply to hairy areas, and they dry rapidly. Patients should be warned that alcohol-based preparations sting on contact with broken skin.

Pharmaceutical manufacturers pay considerable attention to the precise formulation of the vehicle. A topical therapeutic effect of a corticosteroid depends not only on the intrinsic activity of the drug but also on a high bioavailability. Some of the most important recent developments in this respect are the introduction of propylene glycol into ointments as a solvent for the corticosteroid, and the recognition of the effect of urea and salicylic acid as promotors of the penetration of these drugs. They both have a keratolytic effect and enhance the water-binding capacity of the stratum corneum.

The quality of the vehicle also determines the way in which the preparation rubs into the affected skin. This in turn will influence whether the patient will actually use the preparation as prescribed. It is not uncommon to find that a patient has a preference for one particular corticosteroid preparation over others which theoretically have identical therapeutic properties. This may well be attributable to the quality and personal acceptability of the vehicle.

The preservative   A preservative is an agent which inhibits bacterial digestion of the active ingredient – i.e. it prevents the preparation from being degraded once the tube has been opened. Although the specific preservative does not usually influence the physician in the initial choice of a preparation, it may become an important consideration should a patient develop a contact allergy to the preservative. It is usually the preservative that causes such reactions in non-combination topical corticosteroid medications. For this reason manufacturers usually choose a preservative which has a low sensitizing potential. A list of the preservatives used specifically in current topical corticosteroid formulations may be found in the current issue of the *Monthly Index of Medical Specialities* (*MIMS*). This should be consulted if sensitivity to a preservative is suspected.

The topical corticosteroid   The topical corticosteroid is the active therapeutic principle in the formulation. The baseline is hydrocortisone, first introduced into clinical practice over 30 years ago. Hydrocortisone is a very effective agent for many patients with eczema, and provided it is not applied inappropriately to primary skin infections is a very safe treatment with little in the way of side-effects. Modification of the ring structure and side-chains of the corticosteroid molecule, most notably fluorination at the C9 position, have produced a family of drugs with differing therapeutic potencies. It is not of value to list them all, but a full list of those currently available is published monthly in *MIMS*.

It is current practice to classify topical corticosteroids into four classes. The least potent are placed into Class I and the most potent into Class IV (see Figure 2.1). This allows for further classification should a more potent group of corticosteroids than clobetasol propionate become available in the future. There are several ways of assessing the potency of a topical corticosteroid. A generally accepted method is the vasoconstrictor assay. This utilizes the observation that topical corticosteroids induce vasoconstriction within a few hours at the site of application. The degree of vasoconstriction is measured after a standard interval, and this relates to the potency of the preparation.

(a) *Class I – Mildly potent*. These preparations may be prescribed in the long term subject to occasional review. They may be used on the face, for long-term treatment of infantile eczema and for childhood atopic eczema. They are also appropriate for use in the intertriginous areas where the occlusive effect of the tissues and moistness enhance topical corticosteroid penetration and activity. In view of the low incidence of side-effects this group of corticosteroids deserves to be the first choice in the treatment of eczema. Patients who do not respond in the first instance to hydrocortisone, and those who require stronger corticosteroids initially because of the nature of their condition, may be able to return to maintenance treatment with hydrocortisone after some time. There are many proprietary preparations of 1% hydrocortisone available.

(b) *Class II – Moderately potent*. Topical corticosteroids in this group are useful for the long-term management of most types of chronic eczema in adults, but their use on the face and in the intertriginous areas is to be avoided. They also have a part to play in the management of stubborn eczema in childhood but their use must be periodically reviewed. Examples of preparations available are: clobetasol butyrate 0.05%, desoxymethasone 0.05% and fluocinolone acetate 0.00625%.

(c) *Class III – Potent*. A major step forward in the development of topical corticosteroids came in 1964 with the introduction of betamethasone valerate into clinical practice. Class III corticosteroids provide the physician with very effective agents for the short-term suppression of an active eczema. They should not be prescribed for the face, and patients in whom they are prescribed should be reviewed regularly. Other examples of Class III corticosteroids are: desoxymethasone 0.25%, diflucortolone valerate 0.025%, fluocinolone acetate 0.025% and triamcinolone acetonide 0.1%.

(d) *Class IV – Very potent.* Corticosteroids in this group represent the most potent of all the topical agents available, and are invaluable agents for the suppression of very active eczemas, particularly on the palms and soles. They are also particularly useful in the initial management of lichen simplex where less potent corticosteroids seem totally ineffective. Examples of agents available in this group are: clobetasol propionate 0.05%, diflucortolone valerate 0.3% and halcinonide 0.1%.

Mode of action of topical corticosteroids

Although topical corticosteroids have been used for over 30 years the way in which they exert their therapeutic effect is not understood. They have a membrane stabilizing action which may be important. The corticosteroids have an effect on the prostaglandin cascade, presumably through an action of phospholipase A2 which sets in motion the cascade by liberating arachidonic acid from the phospholipid-containing cell membrane. Topical corticosteroids also have an antimitotic effect on the epidermis. This may have therapeutic significance in chronic eczematous conditions in which there is epidermal hyperplasia. The vasoconstrictor effect of topical corticosteroids described earlier may also be relevant to their antiinflammatory effect.

Prescribing topical corticosteroids

A physician must ensure that the treatment is in the right form, and that it contains the most appropriate active ingredient. He must also be able to instruct the patient in how to use the therapy and give advice on possible side-effects.

When treating a patient with eczema the physician must consider the concentration of corticosteroid used, the frequency of application and the total quantity to be prescribed. The duration of long-term treatment must constantly be borne in mind in chronic eczemas.

The corticosteroid preparation of choice is usually the one that contains the least potent agent that is likely to be effective. This depends on the type of eczema to be treated and the site. For example an acute pompholyx eczema of the hands is unlikely to respond to 1% hydrocortisone, whereas a chronic seborrhoeic eczema of the face would be inappropriately treated with a preparation stronger than 1% hydrocortisone. No scientific data exist for the optimal frequency of application of corticosteroids. It is common clinical practice to apply these agents twice daily. Some conditions, however, such as facial seborrhoeic eczema, may require more frequent applications. The quantity of corticosteroid that is prescribed is also important for effective and efficient treatment. It is important to ensure that the patient has sufficient, but at the same time not to be wasteful – potent corticosteroids are expensive preparations. In broad terms 50 g of a topical corticosteroid applied correctly is sufficient for one total-body application of an adult, or twice-daily application to the hands for 2 weeks. If the 'rule of nines' is applied, then 5 g is sufficient for a single application to one 9% area.

Hydration of the stratum corneum caused by occlusion of a topical corticosteroid preparation under polythene gives rise to more rapid penetration and therapeutic efficacy of the drug. Another way to increase the effect of topical corticosteroid therapy is to bypass the barrier effect of the epidermis and inject the corticosteroid into the lesion. Suitable preparations

for this purpose are triamcinolone acetonide and triamcinolone diacetate, which are available in concentrations
from 2.5 mg/ml to 12.5 mg/ml. Care must be taken with this
method of therapy to avoid problems of systemic absorption
and local atrophy.

Side-effects from topical corticosteroids

Side-effects may be systemic or local. Systemic side-effects
come from the use of potent topical corticosteroids for too
long a period of time over a large surface area. It should be
remembered that children have a large surface area to volume
ratio as compared with adults, and are more prone to the
absorption of the corticosteroid.

Systemic side-effects include suppression of the adrenal–
pituitary axis, stunting of growth in children (both from inhibition of growth hormone and epiphyseal closure) and, in
extreme instances, iatrogenic Cushing's syndrome. It is,
however, important that the physician should keep the risk of
systemic side-effects in proportion. Most reported cases of
serious systemic side-effects were caused by carelessly repeated
prescriptions. In adults it requires 100 g per week of topical
corticosteroid of Class III under occlusion or 50 g of a Class
IV corticosteroid to produce significant systemic absorption.
If patients require the use of long-term potent topical corticosteroid then regular estimation of a 9 a.m. plasma cortisol
is recommended. If this is below 150 pg/l then a Synacthen
stimulation test should be performed. In children it is necessary
to ensure that there is no inhibition of growth, by plotting the
height and weight on a percentile chart every 3 months.

In clinical practice much greater problems are caused by the
local side-effects of topical corticosteroid treatment. These
may be listed as follows:

(1) *Skin atrophy*. The skin becomes thin and loses its normal
    elasticity. The underlying veins become easily visible.
    Histologically there is: (i) a marked decrease in the thick-
    ness of the epidermis, and (ii) loss of collagen and ground

substance in the dermis causing atrophy. *Striae* may appear, particularly in the skin folds, as purple linear atrophic lesions. Minor trauma causes *ecchymoses* and extensive lacerations.

(2) *Steroid-induced rosacea.* This occurs, particularly in young women, when an inappropriately strong corticosteroid preparation is prescribed for long periods for minor facial dermatoses.

(3) *Inhibition of melanocyte activity.* This can be a problem in pigmented skins, especially if intralesional corticosteroids are used. Hypopigmentation occurs, which can cause considerable cosmetic distress.

(4) *Allergic contact eczema.* Topical corticosteroid preparations may cause an allergic contact eczema by virtue of the contents of the vehicle, the preservative or, rarely, the corticosteroid itself.

(5) *Glaucoma.* This rare side-effect has been reported from the use of inappropriately potent topical corticosteroid preparations around the eye.

(6) *Spread of infection.* If topical corticosteroids are applied inappropriately to primary fungal infections the condition will spread and change its clinical characteristics – so-called tinea incognito. Application of a topical corticosteroid to primary herpes simplex or bacterial infections may also cause rapid spread of the lesions. This side-effect should be considered in any patient whose condition worsens as the result of application of topical corticosteroids.

(7) *Effects of occlusion.* All the topical side-effects are enhanced by occlusion. In addition specific occlusive effects such as a folliculitis, miliaria and candidiasis can present problems with management.

General guidelines for use of topical corticosteroids

(a) Take care over the initial diagnosis before commencement of therapy. Always consider the possibility of infection with herpes simplex, fungi or primary bacterial infections. If the condition fails to improve reconsider the diagnosis.
(b) Avoid preparations stronger than 1% hydrocortisone on the face.
(c) Avoid potent topical corticosteroids in children.
(d) Avoid the use of potent topical corticosteroids over large areas.
(e) Occlusion enhances the penetration of the corticosteroid. Avoid the use of potent preparations in intertriginous areas.
(f) Use the corticosteroid for as short a time as possible.
(g) Use the weakest corticosteroid that will produce the desired therapeutic effect.

Reducing the strength of a topical corticosteroid

Reduction in strength of topical corticosteroid therapy can be achieved either by reducing to a lower potency class or by diluting the corticosteroid in a given class with an appropriate diluent. It is very important that the diluent is carefully chosen because the wrong choice can significantly affect the bioavailability of the topical corticosteroid. In addition dilution of topical corticosteroids is expensive in pharmacists' time. Therefore it is usually simpler, when maintenance therapy no longer requires a full-strength preparation, to take a formulation from a less potent class.

Use of topical combination therapies

A large number of combination corticosteroids are available. The majority of these are combined with antimicrobial agents, though there are some useful preparations combined with keratolytics and tar.

(i) Combinations with antimicrobials   Examples of the anti-microbials used are given below. A full list can be found in the current *MIMS*.

neomycin (preparations suffixed − N).
tetracycline (preparations suffixed − A).
hydroxyquinolines (preparations suffixed − C).
gentamicin.
imidazoles (e.g. clotrimazole and miconazole).
nystatin.

It is not possible to distinguish entirely between antibacterial agents and antifungal agents as many have activity against both. In general terms, however, neomycin, tetracycline, the hydroxyquinolones and gentamicin are antibacterial. The imidazoles are active against both dermatophytes and *Candida albicans*, whereas nystatin is only active against *Candida albicans*. In all cases it is important to take a swab for culture and sensitivity before these agents are first applied.

At one time, over half the corticosteroid preparations prescribed in the United States were combinations with neomycin. The argument in favour of a corticosteroid–neomycin mixture was two-fold. Firstly, it was felt that an eczema with clinical evidence of infection would clear more quickly if an antibacterial was added to the preparation. Secondly, although many eczemas are not clinically infected they have an abnormally high bacterial count when swabs are taken. In particular, *Staphylococcus aureus* is the dominant organism, and this has been shown to produce potent mediators of inflammation which could potentiate the eczema.

In the 1970s, however, evidence accumulated as to the sensitizing potential of topical antibacterials, and the use of combination preparations has fallen significantly. Another problem encountered with topical tetracycline and the hydroxyquinolones was the staining caused by the preparation. Despite these criticisms many physicians feel it is justified to use a corticosteroid–antibacterial preparation for a short period of 2 weeks to eliminate bacterial growth, but for no longer, to avoid sensitization.

Combinations of corticosteroids with imidazoles and nystatin have an important place in clinical practice. They are particularly useful in the intertriginous areas where secondary candidal infection presents a problem. They do not have great sensitizing potential and do not cause staining.

(ii) Combinations with keratolytics Preparations with salicylic acid and urea are available. These are keratolytic and promote the penetration of corticosteroids into the skin. Salicylic acid also has definite antibacterial and antimycotic properties.

(iii) Combinations with tar A number of preparations combining topical corticosteroids with coal tar distillates are available. The corticosteroid may, in addition to its own therapeutic action, reduce the inflammatory effect of the coal tar and enhance the therapeutic effect.

Systemic corticosteroids

For a severe eczema use of a systemic corticosteroid is justified if there is no immediate response to topical therapy. Systemic agents are also indicated in erythrodermic eczemas. In general they are best used in short courses of between 20 and 30 mg daily for 10–14 days, rather than smaller doses for longer periods of time. Some physicians feel it is safer to use intramuscular injections of depot ACTH. A suitable dosage schedule would be twice-weekly injections until the eczema responds, up to a maximum of 6 weeks.

Systemic antibiotics

Systemic antibiotics should be used if it is considered that infection is playing an important role in maintaining the eczema, or if it has become an important complicating factor.

A swab must always be taken for bacteriological culture and sensitivity before commencing therapy. Until the results of these are available flucloxacillin or erythromycin are appropriate agents. The most common infecting organism is *Staphylococcus aureus*.

Systemic antiviral agents

The possibility of secondary herpes simplex infection must be considered in an atopic individual in whom the eczema is deteriorating. The lesions of herpes simplex are vesicular, as are those of an acute eczematous eruption, and if the patient is not carefully examined the diagnosis may be missed. The clustered nature of the vesicles and central umbilication of the lesions are important diagnostic clues. If in doubt it is better not to apply a topical corticosteroid without antiviral cover because inappropriate treatment of herpes simplex with corticosteroids may lead to life-threatening dissemination of the infection. A swab should be taken for virology and a course of systemic acyclovir given at a dose of 200 mg five times daily for 5 days.

Emollients

The liberal use of emollients is an essential part of the management of chronic eczemas. The emollient should be continued when the eczema has become quiescent, as it will protect the skin against irritants to which these patients are particularly susceptible.

Emollients hydrate the skin surface by applying an occlusive oily film. By hydrating the horny layer the emollient enhances desquamation and decreases scaling and hyperkeratosis. The pliability of the skin is also increased, thus reducing the tendency to fissure. Over and above these effects, the emollients have a mild anti-inflammatory action. They also have mild antibacterial activity. Unfortunately, the effectiveness of emollient preparations is short-lived and they need to be applied repeatedly to have a beneficial effect.

Prescribing emollients

Patients who suffer from a mild dryness of their skin prefer a less greasy preparation than those who have a severe chronic eczema. The use of emollients may be divided into bath additives, soap substitutes and moisturisers.

(a) Bath additives These are added to the bath water and are usually all that is required for a mild dryness of the skin. Patients should be warned that they make the floor of the bath slippery. A variety of proprietary preparations are available and these are listed in *MIMS*. Examples are: Oilatum emollient, Balneum emollient and Emulsiderm which contain lanolin, soya oil and liquid paraffin respectively. Oatmeal is also an effective emollient used either directly or as a colloidal fraction in Aveeno.

(b) Soap substitutes Patients with a dry skin should avoid the detergent effect of soap. They should particularly avoid those with a fragrance, which will irritate their skin. Soap substitutes both cleanse and hydrate the skin. Again there is a large variety of preparations to choose from, but Aqueous cream BP and Unguentum emulsificans (with the optional addition of coal tar as 20% Liquor picis carbonis) are found to be helpful. Unguentum Merck is another useful preparation. Soap substitutes are best applied to the skin and then rinsed off either in the bath or under a shower. Tepid water is to be recommended, and the skin should be patted dry afterwards and not vigorously rubbed with a towel.

(c) Moisturizers Many preparations are available; some of these can be prescribed. It probably does not matter greatly which one is used provided the patient likes to use it and gains some relief from it. Preparations with a fragrance should be discouraged. It is important to prescribe adequate amounts of the moisturizers and encourage patients to apply them

regularly. Aqueous cream BP and Unguentum Merck are suitable light moisturizers; a mixture of 50% white soft paraffin and 50% liquid paraffin is suitable for patients with a very dry skin.

Lotions, Wet Dressings and Soaks

These are water-based preparations and must be applied to the skin regularly. They are used for acute weeping eczemas where their function is to clean and redissolve dry exudate and crust. They also have an antiseptic and astringent action.

(a) Wet dressings Saline compresses can be made by soaking a gauze swab or old cotton sheeting in a solution of normal saline and applying to the affected areas of skin for 20 minutes and then repeating. This is particularly useful for softening crusts to facilitate their removal.

(b) Soaks These preparations are particularly useful for drying out an acute weeping eczema. Potassium permanganate is the most widely used agent. It should be used in a 1 in 10 000 dilution in comfortably warm water. For small areas of skin, such as the hands or lower legs, a bowl or bucket can be used. For more widespread areas the solution can be added to the bath, though this has the disadvantage of staining the bath brown. The preparation is best supplied as a stock solution at a dilution of 1 in 1000, and further diluted by the patient. It is important to explain these instructions to the patient because if it is used as too strong a dilution it has a caustic effect on the skin. The final colour of the solution should be pale pink. Potassium permanganate crystals are also available, but they take a long time to dissolve and it is difficult to make the correct concentration of solution. With an active eczema these soaks may have to be used three or four times daily, reducing the frequency as the weeping subsides. The affected areas of skin should be soaked for 10 to 15 minutes.

Paints

Paints are liquid preparations which are either water- or alcohol-based. They may be applied either with a brush or with a cotton wool bud to the skin. They evaporate and therefore have a cooling effect, as well as being antiseptic and astringent. Alcohol-based paints sting on application to broken skin, and should not be used in an acute eczema.

An 0.5% aqueous Gentian violet paint is a very effective agent for a weeping intertrigo. Its major disadvantage is that it will stain clothing. Care must be taken not to spill the preparation on the furnishings.

Keratolytics

Keratolytics soften keratin and allow for the removal of scale in conditions such as seborrhoeic eczema. They also increase the pliability of the skin and help to prevent fissuring in palmoplantar keratoderma associated with chronic eczemas. The most commonly used keratolytic is salicylic acid, which may be applied in concentrations ranging from 1% through to 10% depending on the clinical situation. Care must be exercised when using high concentrations over large areas to avoid the development of salicylism from systemic absorption of the drug. Urea is another useful keratolytic and is usually used at a concentration of 10% in a cream base.

Shampoos

Shampoos are effectively detergents which clean the scalp and remove scale. Coal tar-containing preparations also have an antimitotic activity and are effective agents in their own right for treatment of scaling conditions of the scalp such as mild seborrhoeic eczema.

Tars

Tars have been used empirically for the treatment of eczemas for many years. The mode of action of tar is unknown, but seems to depend on several of the constituents of the complex mixture of organic substances that is present. Attempts at purification to extract the therapeutically active compounds have not been successful. The tars can be divided by their source into shale, wood and coal tars:

Shale tars – ichthammol.
Wood tars – juniper tar and pine tar.
Coal tars – crude coal tar, coal tar distillate (Liquor picis carbonis).

With the exception of ichthammol-impregnated bandages, the shale and wood tars are rarely prescribed nowadays. Coal tar is still of value in the treatment of chronic eczemas but is no longer indispensable as it was in the pre-topical steroid era. The great drawback of coal tar is that it is messy and smelly. It is also irritant to some individuals and may be a sensitizer for allergic reactions. It can also be phototoxic in some individuals. There are a large number of accepted formulations with coal tar.

Paste Bandages

Paste bandages, consisting of cotton bandages impregnated with pastes, are often overlooked as a means of treating chronic eczemas of the limbs. Pastes are stiff preparations containing a high proportion of finely powdered material. Their use as therapeutic vehicles for the treatment of eczemas has been diminished with the advent of the cleaner topical corticosteroid preparations. However, paste bandages have a dual action in (a) providing a soothing antipruritic effect directly and (b) protecting the affected skin from scratching. Paste bandages are available impregnated with zinc, coal tar, ichthammol and topical steroids. They are applied to the limbs under a retaining bandage.

Systemic Antihistamines

Systemic therapy with a centrally acting antihistamine may be required if the itching disturbs sleep. A suitable preparation is hydroxyzine at a dose of 25 mg nocte for an adult. The use of a sedating antihistamine in children is controversial. There is some argument for the use of trimeprazine, which is available as a syrup, for short periods during exacerbations of the disease. The possibility of a hangover effect and reduced performance at school should be considered. The newer peripherally acting antihistamines are not effective agents for the suppression of itch in eczema.

Environmental Measures

(*a*) *Protection of the skin from irritants*

In patients whose eczema is caused or aggravated by irritants it is important to emphasize the importance of taking protective measures. Many workplaces provide protective clothing, and this should be worn. At present no satisfactory barrier cream has been developed that will protect the skin from irritants. In fact some of those available contain substances which will themselves act as irritants. Non-irritant barrier creams have the advantage of facilitating the removal of dirt and dust, and allow for the use of a less potent and harmful cleanser. The use of emollient creams prior to contact with noxious substances in susceptible individuals may afford some protection as a dry skin is more easily damaged. Application of an emollient after vigorous cleansing is of value.

(b) Removal of an environmental allergen

If a contact allergy is suspected, patch testing should be carried out. This may identify a substance to which the patient is allergic and it is usually a simple matter to exclude this from direct contact with the skin. In some instances, however, the agent is ubiquitous, such as nickel, or cannot be avoided at the patient's place of work. Under the latter circumstance help from the physician in supporting a patient's application for a change in working environment will be helpful.

(c) Dietary manipulation

There is a widespread feeling amongst patients that their eczema is caused by something they are eating. There are very few instances when this can be shown to be the case and where dietary manipulation is recommended. This will be discussed further in the section on atopic eczema, along with removal of other non-food allergens such as housedust mite.

Admission to Hospital

The days when skin wards were full of patients with erythrodermic eczema are now thankfully over. Topical corticosteroids are largely to take the credit for this. However, there are still some individuals in whom topical corticosteroids do not seem to be effective, or in whom the physician is anxious that too potent a preparation is being used for too long. Under these circumstances admission to hospital usually leads to rapid control of the eczema. Admission to hospital is one of the most powerful therapeutic options available. It allows for accurate observation of the patient, gives access to skilled and specialized nursing, provides bed rest and removes the patient from environmental and domestic stress.

Other Forms of Therapy

There are many other forms of therapy that have been used for the treatment of eczema and which have their advocates. Some of these, such as PUVA therapy, will be discussed in the relevant treatment sections.

GENERAL PRINCIPLES IN THE TREATMENT OF ECZEMA

Wherever possible, causative or aggravating factors must be removed. There is little point in prescribing a potent and potentially dangerous treatment when the provoking stimulus is still present. The management of eczema should be based on accurate diagnosis and full assessment of the aetiological factors. In chronic eczemas success often depends as much on the physician's understanding of the patient's personality, social and domestic conditions, and ability to carry out treatments satisfactorily, as on the correct choice of topical medication. Persistent eczema may have caused a fall in living standards through unemployment, causing severe anxiety. The skilful psychological handling of patients is a vital factor in the management of these individuals.

MANAGEMENT OF THE ENDOGENOUS ECZEMAS

Atopic Eczema

Atopic eczema is common, and varies in severity from patients with a rather dry, sensitive, skin to those with severe eczema in whom sleep is disturbed and there is severe disruption of family life.

Support of the family

Reassurance, explanation and encouragement are of great importance in this chronic disorder. Parents of children with atopic eczema need a great deal of support. They often feel guilty about their child having the condition in the first instance, and the parental anxiety is sensed by the child and this seems to aggravate the condition. It is important, particularly in the early stages of management, to give sufficient time for the consultation to allow for adequate explanation of the self-limiting nature of the condition, and what the expectations of therapy should be. The parents should feel that they have ready access to the physician for advice, and that they understand how to use the various preparations that are prescribed.

Self-limiting nature of the condition   Approximately 90% of children with atopic eczema will clear spontaneously and have no active disease by early adult life. It is not possible to predict when they will clear. The skin of these patients remains rather dry, however, and is easily damaged by irritants. For this reason certain careers are not appropriate for atopic individuals.

Careers advice   This is an important part of the management of children with atopic eczema, and should be given early. There is little point in choosing a career that they will not be able to fulfil. Hairdressing, nursing, factory work and car mechanics are not good career choices as they all expose the skin to irritants. This should be made clear to the parents to prevent later disappointments, and they should encourage their children to take up more suitable options.

Clothing   One of the principles of the management of children with atopic eczema is prevention of scratching. Factors known to aggravate atopic eczema should be avoided, such as irritant clothing. Well-washed cotton is the material of choice to wear next to the skin. Wool is to be avoided, as are the rougher synthetic fabrics which do not absorb sweat and further irritate the skin.

Prescribing for atopic eczema

A large number of children with atopic eczema can be treated with emollients alone. Aqueous cream BP is suitable both as a soap substitute and moisturizer.

The aim of treatment with topical corticosteroids is to keep the child comfortable – not necessarily to suppress the eczema completely. This should be explained to the parents. The mildest topical corticosteroid that will keep the child free from scratching should be used. For the majority of children in whom topical corticosteroids are required, 1% hydrocortisone will be adequate. As the skin tends to be rather dry, ointments are generally preferred to creams. Some children, however, are grease-intolerant and find that ointments cause the skin to itch. Also, some children suffer from an occlusion folliculitis if greasy preparations are applied to the skin. Others find that the ointments are just too sticky, and will not use them. Under these circumstances prescription of creams is appropriate.

In more resistant patients with atopic eczema additional measures may be required. The use of more occlusive emollients may be helpful. Unguentum emulsificans (sometimes with additional 20% Liquor picis carbonis) is a very effective soap substitute, though rather messy, and a mixture of 50% white soft paraffin and 50% liquid paraffin is a good moisturizer for very dry skin. It is sometimes appropriate to use more potent topical corticosteroids for a very short period to suppress the more chronic lichenified areas of eczema and then to gradually reduce the strength. Intelligent parents can learn to use three or four different topical corticosteroids at different times or on different sites, provided they appreciate the hazards of using too much steroid for too long. Use of occlusive impregnated bandages, such as zinc and coal tar paste, are very effective for lichenified areas on the limbs. They should be applied at night-time under a retaining bandage. They have a cooling and soothing effect when first applied and they prevent the child scratching the skin whilst asleep. Centrally acting antihistamines may be considered for night sedation for short periods.

If the above measures should fail then the situation must be reviewed. It is important to consider:

(a) whether there is any evidence of secondary infection which requires treatment with a systemic antibiotic;
(b) whether the emollients and topical corticosteroids are being used properly;
(c) whether the child is being irritated by any of the medications, or has developed a contact allergy to one of the components.

If the situation fails to improve then admission to hospital is indicated. Many paediatric wards now have mother-and-child units which reduce the impact of parental separation that was a major drawback to inpatient therapy in the past. For reasons that are not satisfactorily explained children will clear quickly in hospital using the same therapeutic regimen which failed as an outpatient. In some instances it is probable that the parents were simply not applying the preparations, but this does not always appear to be the case. Some argue that removal from domestic environmental factors is important for clearance of the eczema in hospital.

Removal of dietary and environmental allergens

Many parents have been led to believe that food and other allergens play an important role in their child's eczema. Over the past 60 years there have been repeated arguments presented in the literature about the role of food allergens in the pathogenesis of atopic eczema and these are reviewed in Chapter 6. It is probably rare for food alone to be responsible for an individual's atopic eczema. Even if there is a proven allergy it is often more appropriate to consider conventional therapies.

All dietary manipulations are difficult, and should only be suggested when other less uncomfortable measures have failed. The possible benefits of such a harsh regimen must be balanced against the practical aspects of maintaining a diet. It is important for the parents to appreciate that for any diet to be effective it must be absolutely strict. This is relatively straightforward when the child is young and under the parent's direct supervision. As the child grows older, and goes to school, it is not possible for the parents to supervise the diet adequately. In addition the child will already feel different from his peers by virtue of having eczema, and any further measure that will cause further estrangement, such as special diets, will only enhance the feeling of being different and add to the loneliness that affects the lives of many young atopic children. This can only hinder normal psychological development.

There are other factors to be considered when advising parents on the problems of dietary treatment for atopic eczema. It is not possible to predict which children are likely to benefit from a diet. Skin testing and RAST tests for circulating IgE class antibodies to food allergens are unreliable – a positive test does not provide proof that the substance is playing a major role in the child's eczema. Even the history is disappointingly unhelpful. A major difficulty in assessing diets is the great fluctuation that occurs in atopic eczema as the result of the natural history of the disease. This can make historical clues quite misleading.

In severely affected children, in whom there has been no satisfactory response to the general and topical therapies mentioned, there is an argument in favour of a short trial period on a modified elimination diet. Such a diet should exclude dairy products, eggs, chicken, beef, nuts and fruits containing a lot of pips. The eliminated foods can then be reintroduced sequentially at 5–7-day intervals. To be convincing, remissions and exacerbations following dietary withdrawals and challenges must be repeated three or four times at intervals. Very severely affected children in whom there is a firm indication of multiple sensitivities may be considered for a stricter elimination diet – a hypoallergenic diet or an elemental diet. These require the help of an experienced dietician and should not be attempted without this support.

Long-term diets which exclude dairy produce also exclude the child's major source of calcium and an important source of protein. Substitution with goat's milk is not satisfactory as there are cross-reacting antigens with cow's milk. In addition, goat's milk is not generally pasteurized, and carries a high risk of causing an infective gastroenteritis.

Some authorities recommend the use of a soya protein, calcium-enriched, milk substitute but most children find this unpalatable. Although such a substitute may be effective in the short term in children who have a true sensitivity to dairy products, the long-term benefits are not so convincing. Children with atopic eczema are hyperreactive and may eventually develop an allergy to the soya protein itself. One aspect of cow's milk avoidance that has gained widespread acceptance is the benefit of breast-feeding during infancy in children with a strong family history of atopy, although studies on breast-feeding and atopy have shown variable results (Chapter 6).

Some foods appear to cause a widespread erythematous response and may induce a contact urticaria if applied directly to the skin. Animal furs can similarly provoke an urticarial response in some children with atopic eczema. These are not eczematous reactions to the allergen, and do not necessarily mean that the offending agent is causing the eczema. The reaction probably represents the observation that atopic individuals react to a wide variety of foreign proteins. Such allergens are best avoided as they will induce scratching, and this will aggravate the eczema.

There have been some data presented supporting the thesis that non-food allergens such as housedust mite are responsible for atopic eczema. Certainly a proportion of children have a positive scratch test to housedust mite but attempts at exclusion of dust, regular vacuum cleaning, use of linoleum instead of carpets, and plastic coatings on the mattresses, do not constitute practicable advice to give to any but the most obsessional of parents. Desensitization injections to housedust are enthusiastically pursued by some physicians, but the overall results appear disappointing and there is the risk of anaphylaxis.

Alternative approaches

It is a reflection of the failure of good communication with regard to the efficacy and safety of modern corticosteroid-based regimens, rather than the actual failure of these treatments, that has caused some parents to turn to alternative therapies. It is best to keep an open mind about the efficacy of these, but arguments in their favour would be more convincing if the reports were more than anecdotal, and if the methods were subject to the same standard of clinical trial as that required for more orthodox treatments.

The psychological impact of atopic eczema

A child who is severely affected by atopic eczema will suffer considerable psychological distress. Lack of sleep, continuous scratching, repeatedly having to apply topical preparations, being prevented from certain activities such as swimming, will inevitably make him feel different. The other children will tend to shun him and tease him because his skin is different. As a result the child will be tempted to take refuge in his eczema, and may use it in a manipulative way to get what he wants from his fellows. This will cause further resentment. Parents must be given insight into this aspect of atopic disease and be encouraged to make the child take on responsibility for the management of the condition from as early an age as possible. Simple psychotherapy and encouragement are the province of the general practitioner, but severely disturbed children may require specialist psychiatric help.

Treatment of other atopic manifestations of childhood

Lichen striatus   This rare disorder usually remits spontaneously. Application of 1% hydrocortisone cream may be helpful.

Pityriasis alba   This is a distressing condition, particularly on a pigmented skin. It is also self-limiting but most attempts at suppression are unsuccessful. Management consists of explain-

ing the self-limiting nature to the parents, and application of
bland emollients.

Forefoot eczema   Most patients clear spontaneously in due
course. Parents and children should be advised on appropriate
footwear. Trainer-type shoes should be avoided. Cotton socks
should be worn, rather than synthetic fibres which do not
absorb the sweat. If they are affordable, leather-lined shoes or
sandals should be worn; otherwise absorbent insoles should
be used. In severely affected children, with cracking and exudation, bed rest may be needed. A variety of topical preparations   may   help   including   urea   creams,   topical
corticosteroids, Lassar's paste, or coal tar paste, but no single
agent is uniformly helpful.

Atopic eczema in adults

Adults with atopic eczema have a dry skin with intermittently
active eczema. Their eczema may be provoked by extremes
of environmental temperature, low humidity, physical and
chemical irritants or rough clothing. They should be given
advice on avoiding chapping of the skin in the cold weather.

Adults with atopic eczema have usually formed a certain
attitude of cynicism about successfully managing the disease.
This must be countered, and these patients require a great deal
of encouragement and time to explain their treatment. The
same sort of advice is needed as with parents of children with
atopic eczema – they may never have had the treatments
explained to them before.

Exacerbations of atopic eczema in adults may occur for a
number of reasons:

(a)   Secondary infection with bacteria – usually staphylo-
      coccal – or with herpes simplex virus. Widespread herpes
      simplex in an atopic individual is a life-threatening con-
      dition.

(b)   Development of a contact allergic eczema from one of
      the medications. Patch testing is indicated.

(c)   Natural history of the eczema. This can be treated by

use of more effective emollients, more potent topical corticosteroids, use of systemic steroids, or admission to hospital.

Whatever the reason for the deterioration in the patient's eczema he must be reviewed regularly and, should the condition become erythrodermic, referred for urgent admission to hospital. Should the patient be susceptible to regular episodes of severe relapse which require hospital admission a review of the patient's lifestyle is required. There seems little doubt that some individuals are less able to cope with stress than others and a change in occupation may have to be considered.

Other measures for treating severe atopic eczema in adults

Some adults with severe atopic eczema eventually require long-term treatment with systemic corticosteroids. Treatment with PUVA is an acceptable alternative and can be very effective. Its main disadvantages are of regular attendance at hospital for treatment and that high doses of UVA are usually required for control with the long-term possible risk of carcinogenesis. Attempts at immune stimulation with levamisole have not proved helpful and the action of cromoglycate and H_2 antagonists have not been impressive. Some resistant patients have responded to systemic treatment with cyclophosphamide or azathioprine, but these are clearly a last resort.

Seborrhoeic Eczema

Infantile seborrhoeic eczema

This is a self-limiting condition and usually remits by the age of 2. It is important to explain this to the parents.

The scalp should be treated with a mild keratolytic agent. Initially olive oil or arachis oil may be sufficient but if there is extensive cradle cap then a salicylic acid preparation may be required. 0.5% salicylic acid cream is usually adequate. This should be applied at night-time under a cloth bonnet, and washed out in the morning with a mild shampoo. Following this 1% hydrocortisone cream should be applied.

For the body and the face, 1% hydrocortisone cream should be used regularly – up to four times daily if necessary – until the rash comes under control. For the flexures and napkin areas, 1% hydrocortisone with added nystatin to prevent secondary candidal infection should be applied.

Adult seborrhoeic eczema

Adult seborrhoeic eczema is a much more troublesome condition. It persists in varying stages of activity for a number of years. The condition is worse when the patient is tired or under stress.

The scalp can be treated in mild cases with regular daily washing with a coal tar shampoo. There are several on the market and a full list is found in MIMS. Examples are: Polytar shampoo, T-gel shampoo, and Genisol shampoo. It is important to prescribe sufficient for regular use. Some patients are sensitive to coal tar and substitution with a selenium-containing shampoo such as Lenium may be helpful. Otherwise regular washing with Teepol shampoo (Teepol 50%, water 49%, glycerine 1%) may suffice. If this does not prove effective then application of a keratolytic agent is usually effective. A 2% sulphur and 2% salicylic acid cream BNF applied nocte and washed out in the morning with a coal tar shampoo is a suitable regimen. Application of potent topical corticosteroid scalp preparations may be helpful for short periods, but seborrhoeic eczema is a chronic condition and their long-term use is not advised.

The facial rash of seborrhoeic eczema is very responsive to mild topical corticosteroids. It usually settles rapidly with 1% hydrocortisone cream. Patients must be told to apply it initially four times daily and then to reduce the frequency as the condition comes under control. The chronic nature of seborrhoeic eczema must be explained, and that therapy is only suppressive. Otherwise patients will become despondent when the condition relapses, and will lose confidence in the therapy. Should simple 1% hydrocortisone cream fail to suppress the eczema then a combination preparation with a topical imidazole is helpful (e.g. Daktacort, Canesten-HC). The reason for the efficacy of these preparations is not clear, though there have been some reports of *Pityrosporum* species being relevant in the pathogenesis of seborrhoeic eczema in adults. Systemic ketoconazole has also been reported as being effective in controlling severe seborrhoeic eczema, but the condition recurs when the drug is stopped and the potential hepatotoxicity from the drug makes it unsuitable for this disorder.

The body and flexures respond well to application of 1% hydrocortisone cream. A combined preparation with nystatin or imidazoles is indicated for the flexures to prevent secondary candidal infection. The ears are often severely affected in adult seborrhoeic eczema. If there is no response to 1% hydrocortisone, then a combination preparation of a potent topical corticosteroid and antibiotic for a short period may be helpful. Blepharitis is a feature of seborrhoeic eczema and in this situation a topical antibiotic cream (e.g. Albucid) may be effective. Care must be taken, however, not to overlook the sensitizing potential of these preparations. The follicular seborrhoeic eczema that is present over the trunk in some adults is particularly resistant to therapy and potent topical corticosteroids may be required to suppress it. Alternative treatment with long-term systemic tetracyclines may be successful.

Stasis Eczema

Local treatment of this type of eczema will fail if the underlying stasis element is not corrected. The management of stasis eczema must be directed towards controlling the underlying venous hypertension. This may require surgical treatment, and patients with severe stasis eczema should have a surgical opinion. Well-fitting support stockings and adequate firm bandaging from the toes to the knees is necessary. Elevation of the leg for periods during the day is an important part of management and may require supervision by a district nurse, or even admission to hospital.

Topical therapy should be with emollients such as soap substitutes and simple oils such as olive oil, and with mildly potent topical corticosteroid creams and ointments. Potent topical corticosteroids, although effective at suppressing the eczema, may cause atrophy and increase the risk of ulceration. An acute exacerbation may require soaks with potassium permanganate and bed rest with elevation of the leg.

The development of an allergic contact sensitivity may be insidious and the physician should always be on the alert for this. If in doubt, the patient should be referred for patch testing. Topical antibiotics should be avoided because of their great potential for sensitization. Systemic antibiotics may be required if secondary infection with specific organisms is found on culture of a skin swab. The use of fibrinolytic agents such as stanozolol is currently being evaluated. They seem to help with the pain in severely affected liposclerotic legs but they are not without side-effects.

Discoid or Nummular Eczema

An important part of the management of this condition is the avoidance of provoking factors. It is important to use an adequate emollient regimen. Bathing in hot, soapy water with vigorous rubbing with a towel afterwards, degreases and irritates the skin, only to aggravate the condition. Use of fragrances, either in the soap or as bath additives, causes further irritation. To counter this, patients should be advised to take tepid baths only, or better still to take showers. Soap substitutes should be recommended which will hydrate as well as cleanse the skin. Patients should pat the skin dry after bathing rather than risk further injury to the skin by rubbing with a rough towel. Emollients should be applied immediately after bathing whilst the skin is still moist. A potent topical cort-icosteroid may be required initially to suppress the eczema, and ointments are preferable to creams. As the eczema comes under control the strength of the preparation can be reduced. Long-term, regular use of emollients will be required to prevent recurrences. Contributing factors must be explained to the patients, such as low environmental humidity and car heaters. If the discoid eczema fails to respond to this treatment then alternative diagnoses should be considered. Mycosis fung-oides, a cutaneous T-cell lymphoma, can look very much like discoid eczema in the early stages.

Lesions of nummular eczema on the hands

Hand eczema can seriously affect the patient's life. The patient must be instructed in the avoidance of irritants of all types at work and in the home. A list of practical hints is given in the section on irritant eczemas. Small persistent areas respond well to intralesional injections of corticosteroids.

Asteatotic Eczema or Eczema Craquelé

Provoking factors must be removed from the patient's environ-ment. Central heating should be humidified and abrupt tem-perature changes should be avoided. Wool should not be worn next to the skin. Baths should be restricted and should not be too hot. Soap substitutes such as Unguentum emulsificans should be used. A 1% hydrocortisone ointment should be applied three times daily until the eczema is suppressed. Rarely is a more potent corticosteroid indicated if an adequate emol-lient regimen is adhered to. Long-term use of emollients will be required to prevent a recurrence.

Pompholyx Eczema

Pompholyx eczema is difficult to manage. Episodes may take many weeks to settle. In some instances the condition becomes chronic, with hyperkeratosis of the palms and soles and associated cracking and fissuring. In both the acute and chronic forms the condition is incapacitating and may be resistant to all forms of therapy except rest. Pompholyx eczema may be complicated by secondary infection.

Acute pompholyx eczema requires regular, 4-hourly, soaks in a 1 in 10 000 solution of potassium permanganate after the vesicles and blisters have been burst. It will then require the application of a very potent topical corticosteroid cream until the eczema comes under control, reducing to a potent topical corticosteroid cream. Systemic antibiotics may be required depending on the culture and sensitivity results of skin swabs which should be sent regularly. Sedative antihistamines, such as hydroxyzine, 25 mg nocte, are helpful if the patient is unable to sleep. With an acute, severe pompholyx eczema, a short course of systemic corticosteroid is indicated; 30 mg daily of prednisolone, reducing to zero over a 2-week period, should abort an attack.

A chronic pompholyx eczema is characterized by hyperkeratosis and cracking, with the development of painful fissures. It may be particularly severe on the soles of the feet, and may prevent a patient from walking. This condition often responds best to regular use of emollients and keratolytic agents such as 10% salicylic acid ointment or 10% urea cream. The fissures should be protected with Vaseline. Coal tar paste is soothing but patients find it messy. In resistant patients local hand and foot PUVA therapy is sometimes helpful.

Avoidance of irritants is again an important aspect of management of hand eczema. Details are given in the section on contact irritant eczema.

Lichen Simplex or Neurodermatitis

Explanation of the cause of this condition to the patient, together with attempts to break the scratch–itch cycle, form an important part of the management of the condition. Application of a very potent topical corticosteroid may be helpful to suppress itch. Occlusion with an impregnated bandage may be helpful, if the lesions are on the limbs, to prevent scratching of the skin – particularly at night-time when the patient may be unaware that he is scratching. Similarly, systemic, centrally acting antihistamines are of value. A further therapeutic manoeuvre in resistant patients is to inject the lesion with intralesional corticosteroids. Patients should be warned that these injections are painful.

Nodular prurigo is persistent and defies attempts at topical therapy. Some lesions can be injected with intralesional corticosteroids; some respond to occlusion with bandages. In general, however, management is directed towards explanation of the condition and the use of centrally acting antihistamines at night.

MANAGEMENT OF THE EXOGENOUS ECZEMAS

Allergic Contact Eczema

The diagnosis of an allergic contact eczema is suggested by the distribution of the rash. It should always be considered in a patient with an acquired eczema of the face or hands. An idea as to the most likely allergen comes from the combination of a good history and the clinical appearance of the rash. The allergen can be confirmed by patch testing. Removal of the offending allergen should lead to an improvement in the condition. With some allergens which are widespread, careful instructions to the patient as to all environmental sources of the allergen must be given. Some allergens – such as nickel, rubber, perfumes and chrome – are so ubiquitous that complete avoidance is very difficult. Occasionally a change in occupation will be required, and the physician's support in achieving this will be necessary. A contact sensitivity, once acquired, is usually present for the remainder of the patient's life. The patient should also be warned about the problem of cross-sensitivity that occurs with some allergies, e.g. neomycin and framycetin.

The active allergic contact eczema may need to be suppressed with a very potent topical corticosteroid. If the eczema does not respond rapidly to this, allowing reduction to a less potent preparation, then it is probable that the offending agent has not been eliminated completely from the patient's environment.

Irritant Contact Eczema

Many factors contribute to the development of an irritant contact eczema. An atopic constitution, inadequate protection and an underlying dryness of the skin are all important. The strength of the irritant and duration of exposure are both relevant.

The management of an irritant contact eczema consists of minimizing the exposure to irritant substances at home, during leisure activities, and in the workplace. Gloves and other forms of protective clothing should be worn whenever possible. Emollients should be applied to the skin if contact with irritants is anticipated, as this will allow for easier removal of the irritant with less powerful cleansers.

For exacerbations of eczema a short course of a potent topical corticosteroid may be helpful, but this is not recommended for long-term use. In general, avoidance of unnecessary exposure to irritants and regular use of emollients offer the patient the most effective therapy. The following checklist may be of help in giving patients advice on protection from irritants in the home and working environment.

(1) Handwashing – use lukewarm water and avoid the use of scented soaps. Use soap substitutes wherever possible.
(2) Use cotton-lined rubber gloves whenever contact with irritants is anticipated.

(3) Avoid direct contact with detergents (including 'bubble baths') and other strong cleansing agents.
(4) Avoid direct contact with shampoos.
(5) Avoid direct contact with polishes of all kinds.
(6) Avoid direct contact with solvents and stain removers. Do not cleanse the hands with these agents.
(7) Do not peel or squeeze citrus fruits with bare hands.
(8) Do not apply hair creams, hair dye or other hair solutions with bare hands.
(9) Wear gloves in the cold weather.
(10) Do not wear rings for housework – avoid washing the hands with soap when wearing a ring.
(11) The resistance of the skin is lowered for at least 4–5 months after the eczema appears to be completely healed.

Irritant contact eczema in the napkin area in infants requires careful management. The parents must be told the cause, and encouraged to change the nappies as soon as they are soiled. With an acute napkin eczema the infant is often best nursed naked until the eczema has settled – this may require hospital admission. Liberal use of emollients is indicated. Potent topical corticosteroid preparations should be avoided, but weak ones may be used when the condition is acute.

Photosensitive Eczemas

Photosensitive eczemas are caused by a combination of topical (e.g. perfumes) or systemic (e.g. drugs) agents and ultraviolet light. The reaction may be photoallergic or phototoxic. The photosensitizing agent must be identified for effective management of this condition. Sometimes photopatch tests are required. If there is no obvious cause then other causes of photosensitivity should be considered, such as porphyria and systemic lupus erythematosus, and appropriate screening procedures performed.

A sun barrier cream should be prescribed during the acute phase, and the patient should be advised to keep out of direct sunlight. It should be remembered that some sunscreens, particularly the chemical sunscreens such as para-amino-benzoic-acid (PABA), are potential photosensitizers themselves. Physical sunscreens (ROC total sunblock) are also available on prescription.

Suppression of an acute photosensitive eczema may require use of a moderately potent topical corticosteroid agent. In a severe reaction systemic corticosteroids may have to be considered.

MANAGEMENT OF ERYTHRODERMA

Erythroderma, from whatever cause, presents the physician with a serious medical problem. Admission to hospital is indicated for access to skilled nursing care, bed rest, observation and ready availability of laboratory facilities for careful monitoring of the patient's condition. Patients run into difficulties from protein loss, with temperature control and from high-output cardiac failure. If the underlying cause is eczema, patients may require treatment with systemic corticosteroids and bland application of emollient creams.

SUMMARY

The management of eczema can be an immensely rewarding undertaking for the physician. Successful management requires a skilful appreciation of aetiological factors, the psychological impact of the disease and the ability of the patient to carry out the recommended therapeutic procedures correctly. It also requires the physician to be conversant with the wide variety of therapeutic agents that he has at his disposal.

FURTHER READING

Polano, M. K. (1984). *Topical Skin Therapeutics.* (London: Churchill Livingstone

Rook, A., Wilkinson, D. S., Ebling, F. J. G., Champion, R. H. and Burton, J. L. (1986). *Textbook of Dermatology.* (Oxford: Blackwell)

6

THE AETIOLOGY OF ECZEMA

A. V. POWLES

INTRODUCTION

Eczema is a Greek word meaning 'it boils over'. It is thus a descriptive name applied to a particular kind of inflammation of the skin with characteristic clinical and histological appearances. The terms 'eczema' and 'dermatitis' may be regarded as synonymous; the latter is preferred in North America, 'eczema' will be used throughout this chapter.

The *clinical signs* are redness, swelling, papules, vesicles and (rarely) pustules, scaling, exudation of serum, fissures and lichenification (thickening of the skin). In any individually affected area of skin these signs are arranged in a strikingly disordered pattern, often merging gradually into normal skin.

Histological Changes

Whatever the cause of the eczematous process, the histological changes are due to an inflammatory reaction involving both dermis and epidermis. The inflammatory reaction may be severe producing acute eczema, moderate giving subacute eczema, or minimal producing a mild response. Dilation of the capillaries causes redness and exudation into the papillary dermis and spread to the epidermis causes swelling. In the epidermis there is an increase in the intercellular fluid and increase in the intercellular space. If the eczematous reaction is severe there will be damage and eventual destruction of the epidermal cells. Clinically this presents as blisters or an acute weeping area. Whatever the degree of inflammation in the epidermis there is disordered keratinization which in low-grade eczema simply presents as scaling. If the eczema is subacute there will be crust formation which is scale (keratin) and serum together. In chronic eczema with only mild inflammation there is an increase in the number of epidermal cells and increased production of keratin. This results in an increase in thickness of both the cellular component and keratin layer of the epidermis. Clinically this is lichenification. The thickened keratin layer in eczema is abnormal and has a tendency to crack, giving rise to fissures.

GENERAL FEATURES OF ECZEMA

Before considering the classification of eczemas, and the aetiology of the different varieties of eczema, there are several characteristics common to all forms which require explanation.

Itch

While atopic eczema itches severely enough to disturb sleep at times, most eczemas only itch moderately, and some not at all. The threshold for itching on electrical stimulation is fairly constant for any individual at any one time, and varies with the emotional state – lowering of the itch threshold has been used as a measure of stress.

Absence of Scarring

Eczematous skin completely reverts to normal on healing. This means that any anatomical damage is confined to the epidermis.

There are manifold causes (which will be discussed later under individual types of eczemas) for the initial epidermal event which triggers off the process of attraction of lymphocytes and macrophages, which in turn secrete mediators of inflammation to dilate the capillaries in the dermal papillae.

Russell Jones[1] has shown by sequential biopsy studies that the morphological epidermal changes develop only after accumulation of dermal papillary oedema, and that spongiosis appears to reflect the transepidermal elimination of this oedema.

Capacity to Spread

Eczema has a tendency to spread in five different patterns: first by direct extension; but the margin is not sharp as in psoriasis, rather tending to merge into normal skin; secondly indirectly by 'splashes' as it were around the primary patch; thirdly and most interestingly by contralateral spread, from one arm to the same site on the other arm – a mirror-image of the original lesion. In addition to the symmetrical spread from side to side there is also a spread from hands to feet or vice-versa. Fourthly when an eczema is becoming more generalized there is a tendency for it to spread symmetrically to certain areas, e.g. the eyelids, the sides of the face and neck, the flexor (or occasionally the extensor) aspects of the arms and the inner thighs.

Finally eczema may become generalized as erythroderma or exfoliative dermatitis.

Fluctuations and Recurrences

While eczema may persist because the original cause continues
to operate, there is an inherent tendency for eczema to spread,
relapse and recur.

The presence of eczema facilitates the development of
eczema elsewhere. Recently healed eczema relapses in response
to a lesser stimulus than long-healed or normal skin.

The reasons for this general excitation of the skin in eczema,
and this facilitation and habituation of response, are not
known. However, in two varieties of eczema, contact allergic
eczema and atopic eczema, there is recent evidence that activated and memory lymphocytes, and variations in T helper
and suppressor lymphocytes controlling effector lymphocyte
activity, are of fundamental importance in the eczematous
reaction.

The symmetrical mirror-image spread of eczema as yet
eludes explanation. Whether it is related to symmetrical inner-
vation, or whether it is just an identical piece of skin on the
other side of the body with an ability to react to circulating
factors is not known. The tendency for the hands and feet to
react with each other favours the latter theory.

CLASSIFICATION

In the early history of dermatology, when it was a purely
observational art and descriptive science, classification was
based on distinctive appearances and patterns. Different countries and schools produced different names and subdivisions,
resulting in an over-elaborate and confused nomenclature.
Furthermore, two or more forms of eczema may be found at
the same time, or consecutively, in the same patient.

Classification on an aetiological basis has obvious attrac-
tions, and so attempts were made with the terms exogenous,
allergic, seborrhoeic, varicose and neurogenous. Unfortunately, with the exception of exogenous or contact eczema,

the evidence is not enough to maintain this as our aetiological classification.

Eczema is due to the interaction of multiple causes, both exogenous and endogenous. When we use the words 'atopic', 'discoid', 'gravitational' and 'asteatotic' we are describing clinical patterns. But in some of these patterns there is evidence of identifiable and possible aetiological abnormalities.

The latest edition of a major British *Textbook of Dermatology* lists 25 named varieties of eczema. However in considering the aetiology of eczema, those listed in Table 6.1 should suffice our purpose.

Table 6.1 Varieties of eczema

Exogenous	Endogenous
1. Irritant contact	3. Seborrhoeic
2. Allergic contact	4. Asteatotic
	5. Gravitational
	6. Pompholyx
	7. Discoid
	8. Juvenile plantar
	9. Atopic

IRRITANT CONTACT ECZEMA

Irritant contact eczema is five times more frequent than allergic contact eczema. Theoretically any irritant applied in the right concentration frequently enough will penetrate into the epidermis and produce eczema in anyone. An example is the eczema caused by fibreglass spicules. Obviously the efficacy of the skin barrier is the main factor preventing irritant eczema.

The Skin Barrier

The stratum corneum is the principal skin barrier. It can be damaged by repeated minor injuries and lose its protective capacity. It is kept supple by its water content. The preservation of this depends on two factors. First between the epidermal cells are hygroscopic water-soluble cell residues such as urea. Secondly the cells of the stratum corneum are embedded in a lipid matrix and covered by a lipid layer of sebum emulsified by sweat.

The strength of this barrier varies with site, age and predisposition. Thin skin on the backs of the hands and between the fingers, and on the face – particularly the eyelids – is most vulnerable, while palms and soles are most resistant. Babies' skin is more easily damaged, as is fair skin, that of atopics and those with coexistent or recently healed eczema.

Factors weakening the skin barrier   Soaps and detergents and hot water can damage this barrier by dissolving the lipids and washing out the hygroscopic residues (natural moisturizing factors).

Repeated minor damage by both chemical irritants and harmful physical factors such as low humidity, friction, heat, cold and solvents may ultimately break the corneal barrier. Occlusion under rings or straps, rubber gloves, shoes or clothing promotes percutaneous absorption of irritants.

Essential fatty acid deficiency, particularly of linoleic acid, results in increased transepidermal water loss which can be reversed by feeding linoleic acid. Even topical application will lessen the water loss. Other deficiencies, e.g. of vitamin A, vitamin B_2 and B_7 will interfere with the normal maturation of epidermal cells and result in a weakened barrier.

Consequences of skin barrier damage   Once the stratum corneum is breached, and the eczematous process starts, the epidermal cells mature abnormally, producing a defective horny layer which is much more easily penetrated. A great number of normally innocuous substances can therefore perpetuate the injury.

The fine nerve endings in the epidermis transmit the sensation of itch, and are distinct from pain-bearing nerves whose endings are found in the dermis[2]. Endopeptidases from damaged epidermal cells act as a signal to these nerve endings, causing the sensation of irritation resulting in rubbing and scratching, aggravating the epidermal damage and inflammation.

Cumulative irritant eczema (wear-and-tear eczema) is thus the result of a summation of various factors. Eczema results when the repair capacity of the skin is exhausted or when penetration of chemicals damages the living cells of the epidermis and creates an inflammatory response.

ALLERGIC CONTACT ECZEMA

Allergic contact eczema is a Type IV delayed or cell-mediated immunological reaction to penetration of a substance to which the patient has become sensitized.

This type of eczema was first distinguished by Fuchs in 1840 as dermatitis venenata, and considered to be due to an idiosyncratic constitutional predisposition. Jadassholn in 1896 introduced patch tests to identify its cause and showed that related chemicals had a similar cross-sensitization. Bloch in 1911 used *Primula* to produce sensitization in man. Landsteiner in 1936 showed that the simple chemical causing sensitization (hapten) must be combined with a protein to produce this effect, and in 1942 showed that this sensitivity could be transferred by a mononuclear peritoneal exudate from one guinea-pig to another. In 1939 Epstein showed that some chemicals only produced reaction if activated by light. In 1942 Hasthausen proved by transplantation experiments that this reaction was due to a factor supplied to the skin from within.

Frey in 1956 showed that an intact connection with lymph nodes was necessary for sensitization, and in 1974 and 1976 Silberberg showed the importance of Langerhans cells in taking up and presenting the hapten–chemical conjugate to the lymphocyte.

Sensitization

The development of sensitization consists essentially of three stages. First the allergen enters the skin and conjugates with skin protein to form a complete antigen. The allergens in contact dermatitis are of low molecular weight (< 1000 daltons), highly reactive chemically and electron-deficient, capable of forming covalent linkages with protein. However, it is impossible to predict from their chemical configuration (unless they are closely related to known sensitizers) whether any substance will induce sensitivity. Only about a dozen metals have caused contact sensitivity. It is not known why others are harmless in this respect. Secondly the Langerhans cell picks up the complete antigen and possibly migrates to the lymph node where it presents antigen to T-lymphoid cells, specifically activating them against that particular antigen. Alternatively the interaction may take place in the skin and the activated T helper cell migrates back to the lymph node, activating other T lymphocytes there. Some of these lymphocytes then move back to the skin. Thirdly, in a subject thus sensitized, continued or subsequent exposure to the antigen causes the activated lymphocytes in the skin to multiply, producing effector and memory cells, to secrete lymphokines which attract macrophages and activate them for phagocytosis and secretion of inflammatory mediators with subsequent development of eczema at the site of contact.

This sensitization process takes 5 days. With strong sensitizers such as dinitrochlorobenzene (DNCB) a late reaction between 5 and 25 days occurs between the activated T lymphocytes formed and the allergens remaining in the skin. Subsequent exposure to the allergen results in reaction between 8 and 120 hours.

Weaker sensitizers may be tolerated for many years before

contact dermatitis develops, possibly due to impairment of the skin barrier by age or irritants, resulting in a latent sensitivity becoming manifest.

SEBORRHOEIC ECZEMA

This is a distinctive pattern of eczema. The lesions are red, sharply marginated (unlike many other forms of eczema) and covered with greasy scales. They appear in areas richly supplied with sebaceous glands – scalp, face and upper trunk and flexures.

Although common and easily recognized, this pattern of eczema has been bedevilled by the usual confusion of nomenclature and disagreement over aetiology. This suggests that it may be a group of slightly differing reactions to several causes of varying importance in different cases.

Seborrhoea and Seborrhoeic Eczema

The argument has continued for years, but it now seems proved that there is no increased flow of sebum in seborrhoeic eczema, except in rare and atypical cases[3].

Measurements of sebum excretion rate from the forehead of males with classical seborrhoeic eczema prove normal, and in females decreased.

Seborrhoea may occur in Parkinsonism and seborrhoeic eczema may follow. Treatment of Parkinsonism with levadopa reduces excessive sebum excretion and seborrhoeic eczema, if present, often improves. However this might be due as much to the general improvement in well-being as to any reduction in sebum excretion.

A great deal of work has been done on sebum excretion in relation to acne, in which it is definitely increased. There does not appear to be any increased incidence of seborrhoeic eczema in acne sufferers. Suppression of the excessive seborrhoeic

gland activity in acne by means of oral retinoids such as
isotretinoin (Roaccutane) reduces this activity and improves
acne. There is no such evidence of any effect in seborrhoeic
eczema. It therefore appears unlikely that increased sebum
production plays any role in the production of seborrhoeic
eczema.

However, active sebaceous glands appear to be necessary
for the development of seborrhoeic eczema. The sebaceous
glands are active at birth, stimulated by maternal androgen.
When this effect wears off they become inactive until puberty.
The condition known as seborrhoeic eczema of infancy starts
commonly in the early weeks of life after birth, and disappears
usually by the first birthday. Whether it is the same as adult
seborrhoeic eczema is not certain. The latter starts after
puberty, is maximal between 16 and 40 and then declines.

The argument that active sebaceous glands are necessary
for the development of seborrhoeic eczema appears convincing, even though it seems proved that there is no pathogenic
effect from increased activity of these glands. Why sites of high
concentrations of seborrhoeic glands should be involved is not
known.

Infections

It is generally accepted that the lesions of seborrhoeic eczema
show increased colonization by bacteria and fungi, particularly
Pityrosporon ovale, and that the 'seborrhoeic' state is associated with increased susceptibility to pyogenic infections. To
what extent these infections are a cause of seborrhoeic eczema,
or whether they are merely a consequence of the skin changes,
has been disputed for many years.

P. ovale is increased in the scale of dandruff and seborrhoeic
eczema. Kligman suggested that the primary event was
increased cornification and scaling, but Shuster[4], in a critical
review, concluded that *P. ovale* was a causative agent. This
opinion was supported by the finding that oral ketoconazole,

active against fungi, improved dandruff and seborrhoeic eczema[5]. Unfortunately ketoconazole was later found to have potential serious side-effects, making its use for the purpose undesirable. How *P. ovale* may cause seborrhoeic eczema is unknown. It may theoretically do so by activating complement to induce inflammation.

Hypersensitivity to bacteria, particularly staphylococci, may be a cause in some cases. The observation that it is common in the acquired immunodeficiency syndrome (AIDS)[6] suggests that reduced immunity to infection may be an aetiological factor.

Certainly there is an increased susceptibility to bacterial infection and to physical and chemical injury, so that seborrhoeic subjects may frequently exhibit contact and infective dermatitis.

Stress

There is no doubt that stress, whether physical or mental, will aggravate seborrhoeic eczema. Lack of sleep, jet-lag, surgical operations, and other illnesses will exacerbate or precipitate this type of eczema. Stress alters the circulating levels of certain hormones including cortisol, which may have an effect on eczema, or it may be mediated via the hormonal effects on the immune system.

To summarize, there appears to be a constitutional predisposition, and infection, stress and fatigue precipitate attacks.

INFANTILE SEBORRHOEIC ECZEMA

This is a distinct pattern of infantile eczema and has been differentiated from atopic eczema because of its earlier onset, the lack of itching (a baby with seborrhoeic eczema is generally happy and cheerful, unlike the misery and restlessness of the baby with atopic eczema), the absence of stigmata of atopy, the predisposition for the scalp and intertriginous areas, the well-circumscribed lesions and the good prognosis. However, it has been argued[7] that it is just a variant pattern of atopic eczema with a different prognosis. More recently one study showed that children with seborrhoeic eczema in infancy had a higher than normal incidence of atopic manifestations 15 years later, suggesting that infantile seborrhoeic eczema may be part of the spectrum of atopic disease[8].

Although the intertriginous lesions may suggest a candidal infection positive cultures are only found in 25% of patients.

Infantile seborrhoeic eczema of the napkin area looks psoriaform (lesions of seborrhoeic eczema and psoriasis may at times be difficult to distinguish clinically in adults as well as babies). However it is rare for these children to develop psoriasis later, and HLA studies show no increase in frequency of B13, B17 and BW37 in children with so-called napkin psoriasis, while they are significantly increased in true psoriatics.

As in adult seborrhoeic eczema, there is a constitutional or genetic abnormality which may or may not be related to atopy, resulting in seborrhoeic areas of the skin being vulnerable to irritants and infection, more liable to react by inflammation in an eczematous form.

ASTEATOTIC ECZEMA (ECZEMA CRAQUELÉ)

'Asteatotic' means without fat, and this form of eczema is associated with, and may be due to, a decrease in skin surface lipids.

Loss of surface lipids will lead to an increase of water loss from the epidermis. The transpiration rate of fluid through the skin is dependent on the lipid layer. Experiments on excised skin have shown that if the lipid layer is removed water loss increases 75 times, and restoration of the lipids reduces the loss to normal levels. Loss of water from the epidermis will predispose to damage to the stratum corneum and therefore precipitate eczema.

The factors concerned with this development of asteatotic eczema appear to be a naturally dry skin with a tendency to chapping; a reduction of skin lipids from age and hormonal decline, illness or malnutrition; increased transpiration of water; damage to the water-containing stratum corneum by domestic or industrial detergents; low humidity, cold drying winds increasing heat loss; repeated minor trauma leading to inflammation and increased percutaneous absorption of irritants and sensitizers.

For years patients vulnerable to this condition may simply complain of dry skin and chapping in the winter. Eventually, some minor additional insult may turn the scale. In industry, after years of contact with degreasing agents, a sudden disabling eczema may arise, or retirement with extra gardening and unaccustomed manual work, a particularly bitter winter, or the installation of central heating may provoke the eczematous change. Bubble baths (which are detergents) seem to be an increasing cause of asteatotic eczema.

GRAVITATIONAL ECZEMA

This is the preferred term for eczema of the lower leg related to venous hypertension. Formerly it was called varicose or stasis eczema. However, varicosities may be present without eczema, and they are not essential for the development of the condition. Furthermore, the venous blood in such limbs has a faster circulation time than normal and the oxygen content of the femoral venous blood is increased.

Venous hypertension may be the result of deep-vein thrombosis. Localized venous hypertension may occur due to incompetence of the valves of perforating veins connecting the deep and superficial venous systems, and an incompetent perforating vein can often be palpated under a patch of gravitational eczema.

Browse and Burnand[9] have suggested that high venous pressure is transmitted to the capillary circulation in the skin and subcutaneous tissues, distending the capillaries and widening their endothelial pores. This allows fibrinogen molecules to escape into the interstitial fluid and form fibrin cuffs around the capillaries. This thick fibrin cuff impedes the diffusion of oxygen and nutrients to the skin, resulting in devitalization, damage and eczema. However the exact mechanism, as to how these events cause eczema, remains obscure.

This fragile skin is more vulnerable to all the exogenous causes of eczema – chemical and physical irritants, drying, rubbing and scratching, infection and contact dermatitis, especially from medicaments.

POMPHOLYX

Pompholyx (vesicular eczema of the palms and soles or dyshidrotic eczema) means a bubble, cheiropompholyx refers to the palms and pedopompholyx to the soles. Because it was thought to be due to blocked sweat ducts at one time the other term was dyshidrotic eczema. However it has been shown that the 'bubbles' lie between, not in, the sweat ducts. They are formed under the thick corneum of the palms and soles by vesicles coalescing to form bullae, rather than bursting and releasing exudate. The aetiology of this form of eczema is again obscure, although emotional tension and heat have been implicated.

The role of hereditary and atopic eczema may be relevant. There have been reports of up to 30% of a personal or family history of atopy occurring in patients with pompholyx eczema. There may be a higher incidence in the spring, and this is possibly related to the hayfever season. Skin tests to pollen have shown a higher incidence of positive reactions, as have skin tests for housedust and human dander, but this may be a reflection of an underlying atopic state, rather than being of aetiological significance.

The role of excess sweating is not clear. Hyperhidrosis does seem to be a feature in some patients, particularly those with small 'sago-like' vesicles along the sides of the fingers, and is more common in hot weather.

Nickel allergy has also been implicated, as have other allergens including cobalt, chromate and perfume. In chronic pompholyx eczema it has been suggested that patch tests should be carried out[10]. However, even if patients are nickel-sensitive, the value of nickel avoidance and low-nickel diets have not proved beneficial in the majority of patients.

ID REACTIONS

The term 'id' was used to denote a reaction to a primary focus, e.g. eczematide for an eczematous reaction to a disorder elsewhere in the skin. In the days when a 'toxic focus' was the medically popular explanation for any illness whose cause was unknown, the terms toxic bacteride and dermatophytide were much used.

Dermatophytides (i.e. an eczematous reaction at a distant site from a fungal infection) undoubtedly occur. To prove the diagnosis fungus must be cultured, usually from the feet, and the id reaction (usually on the palms) must respond to clearing of the foot fungal infection by a fungicide. Dermatophytides are not as common as pompholyx affecting both the hands and feet.

Pustular toxic bacteride may possibly occur, but is difficult to prove. Many cases thus diagnosed in the past later proved to be pustular palmo-plantar psoriasis.

Irritant or allergic contact eczema of the feet can also give rise to an id reaction of the palms (eczematide). In this context it must be emphasized that the skin generally is hyper-irritable in the stage of active eczema. In patch testing this is known as the 'angry back' phenomenon. This hyper-reactive skin results in the spread of eczema, and has been termed 'autosensitization', and in its severest form will lead to erythroderma (generalized eczema).

DISCOID ECZEMA (Nummular Eczema)

This condition is characterized by discoid lesions of eczema. The aetiology is unknown; there have been many theories put forward, none of which has been proven. The condition is rare in children but it can occur in association with atopic eczema. In adults the association with atopic eczema is less obvious and the level of IgE is usually normal. Various precipitating factors have been reported, and these include emotional stress, infection, local physical and chemical trauma, food allergy and specific contact allergic sensitivity. Sensitivity to nickel, and also to cobalt, has been found in patients on patch testing. Drying out of the skin by central heating and detergents is also said to account for the recent increase in incidence.

JUVENILE PLANTAR ECZEMA

This variety of eczema has been described only since 1968[11]. It is attributed to the use of synthetic materials for socks and footwear, and is particularly associated with 'Trainers'. These materials are less porous than those they replaced, and a repellant coating to improve durability increase this effect. Thus the feet are subjected to hot humid conditions resulting in maceration and sweat retention.

This is only part of the story. The condition is practically never seen in pre-school children or adults, and is commoner in children keen on sports. Friction therefore probably also plays a part.

There is disagreement over possible association with atopy. Atopic subjects probably have a more vulnerable skin with a lower threshold for damage.

ATOPIC ECZEMA

The term atopy (a Greek word meaning different or strange) was coined by Coca, an allergist at Columbia University in 1923. He used it to describe a form of sensitivity based on hereditary influences in asthma and hayfever, and later included atopic eczema in this group.

In 1933 Wise and Sultzberger suggested atopic 'dermatitis' to cover the whole spectrum of atopic skin disease from the weeping eczematous lesions to the later dry lichenified form.

Atopic eczema is the commonest form of eczema in children, affecting about 3% of all infants.

Research into aetiology is hindered by the lack of a distinct objective diagnostic indicator. It is still a clinical diagnosis. There are probably subgroups of atopic eczema which are distinct genetically and biochemically.

Itch

The fundamental basis appears to be a constitutional pre-disposition to develop pruritus. The itching leads to scratching, skin trauma and eczema. The following statements have been made emphasizing the importance of itch in atopic eczema: (a) 'it is not the eruption which itches but the itch which is eruptive'; (b) 'If the fingers of a patient with atopic eczema could be restrained the skin lesions would disappear, although the itching would doubtless persist.'

Areas of atopic eczema itch more readily and more easily with stimuli which normally cause itching, e.g. histamine, and also respond with sensation of itch to stimuli normally felt only as touch, e.g. woollen clothing. The patient judges the severity of his condition not by the appearance of his skin but by the intensity of the itch. In general if a rash does not itch it is unlikely to be atopic eczema.

Itch and Late Cutaneous Reactions

In atopic eczema not only does itching appear 15 minutes after allergenic challenge, e.g. with a known allergen, but new waves of itching occur after 4–6 hours which can last until 24 hours after challenge. After 4–6 hours a mild pruritus is followed by an exacerbation of inflammation which peaks at 6–12 hours. At the height of the response the lesion is characterized by erythema, warmth, pruritus and/or tenderness, much more extensive in area and producing greater discomfort than the initial wheal-and-flare response.

This is the late cutaneous reaction, or late phase of immediate-type reaction, and is due to release of chemotactic mediators, and possibly histamine, from the surface of mast cells or basophils during an IgE–anti-IgE reaction.

This may be the explanation of the peculiar spreading itch which is so characteristic of atopic eczema.

Itch and Histopathology

Recently, in addition to the normal changes of eczema, increased mast cells, prominence of superficial venules, demyelination and perineural fibrosis of dermal nerves in affected and unaffected skin has been observed[12]. These changes, not observed in contact eczema, may be peculiar to atopic eczema and of significance in relation to the pathological itching characteristic of the disease.

Hereditary Factors

About 70% of patients with atopic eczema have a family history of atopy, if one includes the three major atopic disorders – asthma, allergic rhinitis and atopic eczema. Those patients without a family history do not differ clinically from the rest. Clinically normal parents may have affected children, and in other families both parents may be affected while the children are normal. Inheritance, therefore, cannot be due to a simple dominant or recessive gene.

It has been postulated that the principal atopic gene is an autosomal dominant with low or variable penetrance. If this is so, it will not infrequently fail to express itself in recognizable clinical abnormality, and consequently isolated non-familial cases can be expected to occur regularly. These non-familial cases may be assumed to have a hereditary predisposition. That latent atopy can exist is well shown in studies of identical twins.

Whether the atopic gene is pleiotrophic, predisposing to both skin and respiratory disease, or whether the various atopic manifestations are expressions of different genes is not yet known. The evidence suggests that a 'principal' gene is responsible for the manifestations of atopy, and a different gene determines whether skin disease occurs, and that the inheritance of atopic eczema is polygenic.

Physiological and Pharmacological Aspects

The inherent irritability of the skin may be related to certain physiological and pharmacological vascular peculiarities found in atopics.

The small blood vessels have a tendency to vasoconstriction, especially on exposure to cold. The atopic tends to have cold hands and pallor especially around the nose, mouth and ears. He or she may show white dermatographism – blanching at the site of trauma. The speed of the response suggests vasoconstriction. Following intradermal injection of acetylcholine an area of blanching spreads around the red flare, and following the inunction of tetrahydrofurfuryl nicotinate (Trafuril) pallor develops instead of erythema. The pallor may be due to capillary vasoconstriction, or to capillary dilation and oedema.

Acetylcholine   The paradoxical white reaction that follows intradermal injection of acetylcholine is evidence of atopic hyper-reactivity to cholinergic agents, also shown by an increased incidence of cholinergic urticaria and an increased eccrine sweat response. Acetylcholine levels in skin of atopic eczema subjects have been reported to be 15 times higher than normal. A pathological role for acetylcholine in atopic eczema has been suggested, regulating and even stimulating histamine release, and also abnormal cholinergic neurotransmission may be involved in the lowered itching threshold.

Histamine   Hyper-reactivity to histamine is a feature of all forms of atopy. In atopic eczema intramuscular injection of histamine showed greater erythema over the face, neck and flexures than in normals. Increased skin histamine levels even in uninvolved skin have been noted, and transiently elevated plasma levels in severe cases of atopic eczema.

Basophils in atopic subjects have a lowered threshold for histamine release, i.e. anti-IgE-induced histamine release is higher in atopic eczema children than controls. Mast cells and basophils release mediators more easily in atopic eczema. These findings are consistent with defective mast cell and basophil control mechanisms. Many features of the disease may be related to excess blood and tissue histamine.

Immunological Factors

Reaginic allergy and atopic eczema

The association with asthma and allergic rhinitis originally suggested that atopic eczema might likewise be caused by reactions between antigens and tissue-fixed reaginic anti-bodies.

The reaginic antibody that mediates most anaphylactic

(immediate) allergic reactions was identified as immuno-globulin E (IgE) by Ishizaki in 1966. It is formed by atopic persons to a wide variety of common environmental allergens. These are inhalants, foods and micro-organisms, and it was noted that there was a similarity in their chemical structure and molecular weight.

Patients with atopic eczema show a high incidence of positive scratch (prick) tests to these allergens (up to 80%). However, the lesions of atopic eczema are not urticarial wheals of Type I hypersensitivity, nor any other of the four recognized types of immune reaction. Moreover, many years of skin testing have shown that it is of little value in eliciting the aetiology of atopic eczema. The patient's history is of much more importance, identifying possible allergic causes, although positive skin tests may confirm the atopic state and possibly predict respiratory atopic disease[13].

About 82% of patients with atopic eczema have been shown to have elevated serum IgE levels, and a relationship between IgE levels and the severity of the eczema has been demonstrated. However, it is unlikely that an antigen–IgE–mast cell mechanism is a primary cause of atopic eczema for the following reasons:

(1) Elevated serum IgE levels are found in non-atopics following injections of vaccines, e.g. tetanus, or as a result of parasitic infection.
(2) Serum IgE levels remain high in remissions of atopic eczema, only falling after prolonged disease-free periods.
(3) Atopic eczema occurs in patients with low or absent serum IgE, particularly those with pure atopic eczema (i.e. without allergic respiratory disease), and those with agammaglobulinaemia.

Thus elevated serum IgE is a non-specific feature of atopic eczema, possibly a sign of a more basic derangement of control mechanisms that regulate immunoglobulin production. However, this does not preclude IgE being a mediator in the pathogenesis of the eczematous process.

Possible causes of raised IgE levels

Since increased serum IgE is a feature of atopic eczema, search for the mechanism involved may give clues to the aetiology of atopic eczema.

Lack of T suppressor cells   In atopic eczema T suppressor cells are diminished[14], and it has been shown that there is an inverse relationship between serum IgE levels and T suppressor cells[15]. B cells, which are under the control of T cells, from atopic individuals have shown increased production of IgE in culture[16]. Co-culture experiments of normal and atopic T and B cells have yielded inconsistent results, suggesting that in some patients T cells may be defective whilst in others B cells are abnormal. Thus the immunological abnormality may be of a more general nature than related to a specific cell line.

Lack of IgA   IgA is the normal immunoglobulin produced by the intestinal mucosa to protect the body against foreign protein. Secretory IgA found on the surface of the epithelium binds to the foreign antigen and is shed with the antigen. IgA production does not begin until the age of 3 months and it has been claimed[17] that in children of atopic parents, who subsequently develop atopic eczema, there is a relative deficiency of IgA at the age of 3 months in these individuals. IgE antibody response occurs to the foreign antigens, and not IgA, and this leads to sensitization. IgE antibodies are not eliminated from the surface of the intestine as occurs with IgA. Once sensitization occurs the process appears to be self-perpetuating for many years, and leads to high levels of IgE. Since atopic eczema does not start until after 2 or 3 months of age, some neonatal defect such as lack of secretory IgA predisposing to early antigen exposure and excessive IgE formation is an attractive hypothesis, and may be aetiologically important in some patients.

Relative increase in dermal T helper cells

Cyclosporin A, which is known to have a specific effect on T helper cells, is being used to treat psoriasis which is thought to be a T helper cell-mediated disease. Cyclosporin has also been used to treat severe atopic eczema successfully. This is likely to be due to its effects on T helper cells, a high ratio of T helper to T suppressor cells has been found in the dermis of active lesions of atopic eczema[18]. This exceeds the increased circulating T helper to T suppressor cell ratio in this disease. These observations suggest that atopic eczema is also mediated by T helper cells.

Cyclic AMP and cyclic GMP

In intracellular metabolic reactions of oxidation or dehydrogenation the energy produced is not all dissipated as heat, but some is banked in high-energy phosphate compounds from which it can later be released by enzymes to effect chemical synthesis and to perform work, e.g. secretion.

One of these systems consists of the enzyme adenylcyclase found on the inner surface of the cell membrane. Adenylcyclase, when activated by an appropriate extracellular stimulus, forms cyclic adenosine monophosphate (cAMP). This in turn is inactivated by the enzyme phosphodiesterase. Intracellular cAMP is the resultant of the rate of formation by adenylcyclase and inactivation by phosphodiesterase.

Another linked system consists of guanylate cyclase which increases cyclic guanosine monophosphate (cGMP). cAMP and cGMP have opposite effects on antigen–IgE interactions. When antigen combines with two adjacent molecules of IgE on the surface of the mast cell, causing release of histamine and other mediators, cGMP enhances (and cAMP inhibits) movement of mast cell granules along microtubules, fusion of granule membrane and cell wall and secretion of histamine, by exocytosis. So beta-adrenergic drugs, e.g. isoprenaline, which stimulate adenylcyclase and so cAMP formation, will lessen

the production of histamine from mast and basophil cells, and
beta-blockers will have the reverse effect. Acetylcholine also
increases the production of histamine, not by decreasing intracellular cAMP but by stimulating guanylate cyclase and
increasing cGMP.

Local steroid application may theoretically exert a beneficial
effect in atopic eczema, not only by the local vasoconstriction
they produce, but also by their ability to stimulate adenylcyclase and thus cAMP, reversing the imbalance between
cAMP and cGMP which is a possible biochemical mechanism
underlying atopic eczema.

Low levels of cAMP have been reported in leukocytes in
atopic eczema[19], and this has been taken to imply altered
response to chemical mediators. Whether this reduction of
cAMP is a primary or secondary event remains to be determined.

Beta-adrenergic blockade and desensitization

Szentivanyi proposed the beta-adrenergic blockade theory in
1968[20] to explain some of the alterations in pharmacological
reactivity observed in atopics. A reduction in beta-adrenergic
receptors, damage from autoantibodies, a qualitative abnormality or alternatively a relative increase in alpha-adrenergic
receptors has been postulated. Responses to catecholamines,
such as constant pilo-erection in the skin of atopics, decreased
phenylephrine threshold for pupillary dilatation and
cutaneous vasoconstriction, gave support to the theory. Much
of the work in relation to beta-adrenergic responses had been
carried out using leukocytes from atopic eczema patients and
comparing these to cells from normal individuals. Leukocytes
from atopic patients showed decreased production of cAMP
in response to beta-agonists, but also to histamine and prostaglandin E. This suggested that the defect was not confined
to the beta-receptor.

Incubation of normal leukocytes with low concentrations
of isoprenaline, histamine and prostaglandin E causes 'desen-

sitization'. These cells then behave like atopic leukocytes in that stimulation with any of these agents produces subnormal cAMP responses. Histamine desensitizes within 15 minutes, and recovery takes place over 3–4 days. The desensitizing concentration of histamine is similar to that found in the plasma and skin of atopics. This *in vivo* level of histamine in atopics may render cells less responsive to catecholamines and other agonists which normally regulate their function via cAMP.

Normal cells exposed to desensitizing concentrations of histamine, isoprenaline or prostaglandin E develop increased cAMP phosphodiesterase activity. This could explain the decreased cAMP levels in these cells after agonist stimulation as being due to increased breakdown rather than decreased production. Leukocytes from atopic eczema patients have consistently elevated phosphodiesterase activity, which would further suggest desensitization as a mechanism for the beta-blockade theory. Elevated phosphodiesterase activity, with its resultant decreased level in cAMP responses in basophils and mast cells, could explain the increased histamine releasability in atopic eczema.

Cell-mediated (delayed) immunity in atopic eczema appears to be reduced or defective. While contact allergy does occur in these patients, the incidence is lower than normal. Sensitization to strong allergens such as poison ivy and dinitrochlorobenzene (DNCB) has a low incidence. Depressed responses to tuberculin have been noted, and the depression varies with the severity of the eczema.

The depression in delayed reactivity to infectious agents in atopic eczema is well documented. Kaposi in 1895 first described the susceptibility of these patients to unusually severe cutaneous infections with vaccinia and herpes simplex viruses. There is an increased incidence of prolonged infections with warts, molluscum contagiosum and cutaneous fungal infections.

This hyporeactivity is thought to be due to lymphocyte functional defects of T cells, resulting in impaired mobilization of leukocytes, impaired activation of the monocyte–macro-phage system, reduced chemotaxis, and reduced antibody-dependent monocyte-mediated cytotoxicity.

Bacterial Infections

Impaired resistance to infection suggests that bacteria may be responsible for the lesions of atopic eczema. The improvement in some patients with the addition of an appropriate antibiotic to their existing treatment is suggestive evidence. The bacterial flora of eczematous lesions is greatly increased, and though bacteria of several genera and species occur on the skin those most frequently colonizing it are staphylococci. This may be due to the damaged skin barrier, scaling and exudation providing a more hospitable field for the staphylococci to multiply. However the unaffected skin of eczematous patients carries more *Staphylococcus aureus* than does skin of normal persons[21].

The demonstration that organisms are present does not establish that they are the cause, or even altering the lesions, and a distinction must be made between colonization even at a high level, and infection. However, clinical infection is not uncommon in atopic eczema, and an impaired neutrophil chemotaxis has been demonstrated in some cases[22].

Bacterial antigens can promote a cytotoxic reaction in the skin. Bacteria dying in the stratum corneum release soluble antigen, some of which diffuses into the epidermis and becomes firmly absorbed to the epidermal cells. Antibacterial antibody and complement diffusing into the epidermis react with the antigen acquired by the cells, and may induce lysis. Endo-peptidases released from damaged skin cells and bacteria can stimulate nerve endings in the epidermis to cause itching. As this cytotoxic reaction depends upon the greatly increased growth of bacteria in the skin, and upon the increased vascular permeability predisposing to epidermal diffusion of anti-bacterial antibody, the reaction is only likely to occur in skin that is already damaged[23]. In acute eczema the skin is moist because of exudation due to increased vascular permeability. Hydration of the epidermis, particularly the corneal squames, provides optimal conditions for growth of bacteria abundantly present on eczematous skin. Therefore it seems likely that bacteria may aggravate and perpetuate atopic eczema, but that they do not initiate the condition. This is further supported by a double-blind study[24] that showed that mupirocin, an effective topical antibiotic against *Staphylococcus*, was effective in clearing the bacteria but was not associated with any difference in the rate of improvement or subsequent relapse of the eczema.

Allergens

Atopic diseases are often thought to result from early antigen exposure of genetically susceptible individuals who are unable properly to control IgE synthesis. How true this is of atopic eczema has been, and continues to be, a matter of dispute.

Inhalant allergens

Pollens, animal hair, human dandruff and housedust mite, moulds and algae have all been found to give positive skin tests in a small percentage of patients, but the evidence that they play any aetiological part is unconvincing. For example IgE does not increase in 'pure' atopic eczema in the pollen season[25].

However Mitchell et al.[26] have shown that an inhalant allergen (housedust mite extract) when *applied* under occlusion to mildly abrased *skin* of subjects with severe atopic eczema, and positive skin tests to housedust mite, would give rise to eczematous reactions. Repeated applications for some days resulted in a mast cell hyperplasia replacing the earlier basophil infiltration, thus resembling the chronic lesions of atopic eczema.

Food allergens

Some patients with atopic eczema undoubtedly have food allergies which exacerbate their disease. Because of the difficulty in obtaining reliable evidence there is disagreement over the number of patients affected, and the frequency of relevant food-induced flares of eczema.

Food allergy as a cause of atopic eczema has been a theory more popular with the general public and doctors in other branches of medicine than with dermatologists. Possibly the latter tended to see patients in whom food exclusion had failed to improve atopic eczema. One study[27] found that exclusion diets based on the results of skin tests gave poor results. Agreement between food ingestion challenge tests and skin tests was poor. The clinical history and skin tests only weakly correlated. RAST (radio-immunological allergen-specific–IgE *in vitro* assay test) offered no advantage either alone or in combination with skin testing, for evaluation of food hypersensitivity in atopic eczema.

Breast-feeding

If lack of IgA is of aetiological importance in the development of atopic eczema, then breast-feeding should decrease the chance of its development, particularly since breast milk contains much secretory IgA. The other obvious benefit of breast-feeding is that food antigens are given later to the infant when the immune system may have matured sufficiently to handle them.

However, it is difficult to find evidence that breast-feeding protects against the development of atopic eczema. One study[28] even suggested that there was a higher incidence of atopic eczema in breast-fed children. In this particular study the diagnosis of 'eczema' was made from clinic records, from health visitors' observations and from recollections of mothers 7 years later. All that in fact it showed was that 'eczema' of any sort – atopic, seborrhoeic, ichthyotic, even nappy rash –

was reported more often and remembered better by mothers who breast-fed. Other studies have also shown no advantage prophylactically from soya or breast-feeding[29].

It is always difficult to be sure that a breast-fed baby has not occasionally had cow's milk preparations. It has also been suggested that the mother's diet is important, and that egg and milk she consumes may result in allergens from these substances being passed on to the baby in her milk.

Food Exclusion and Challenge Studies

Most of the older studies were so flawed in design that their conflicting results were useless. However in the past 10 years two or three impressive studies have suggested that food hypersensitivity may be more common and relevant than previously realized. Atherton et al. in 1978[30], by a double-blind controlled crossover trial, showed that a diet excluding common food allergens, e.g. milk and eggs, resulted in an improvement in many but not all cases. Matthews et al.[31], the previous year, reported that the elimination of common food allergens in the first 6 months of life in high-risk infants reduced the incidence of eczema but not consistently, though complete avoidance was difficult.

Sampson[32] studied 26 children with atopic eczema and histories of possible food allergies. They were tested in hospital by double-blind challenges. None of the 104 placebo challenges was positive. Twenty-three of 104 food challenges were positive in 15 of the children, producing cutaneous erythema and pruritus within 15 minutes to 2 hours after challenge. Among positive food challenges 36% were to egg, 14% to milk, 11% each to wheat and peanut, with other reactions to soya, chicken, fish, chocolate, potato and rye. Most of the children showing food sensitivity gained marked improvement by strict avoidance of offending foods, though none cleared completely.

Some earlier studies have shown that the rapidity of the cutaneous reaction is related to the increased intestinal permeability for high molecular weight reagents in patients with atopic eczema, either as a primary defect or as a consequence of local hypersensitivity reactions[33]. Other studies have not shown an increased intestinal permeability.

The food antigens may be delivered directly to cutaneous mast cells sensitized with specific IgE, triggering mediator release, or circulating complexes might iniate reactions.

Food allergens thus, in some cases – particularly in children – cause an immediate skin reaction both with ingestion and with skin contact, as Pike and Atherton described with egg white on susceptible infants' cheeks[34].

SKIN ABNORMALITIES IN ATOPIC ECZEMA

The immunobiochemical changes so far described act on an abnormal skin to cause itch and skin alterations of atopic eczema. More than 50% of atopic patients have dry skin, and almost 50% of patients with autosomal dominant ichthyosis have some evidence of atopy.

The number of sebaceous glands per skin area is reduced in atopic eczema, and sebum secretion is often reduced, with the result that transepidermal water loss is increased. The dry scaly skin of atopics leads to impaired barrier function and an increase of colonization with staphylococci. This dry skin is particularly vulnerable to the external factors shown to be the cause of irritant eczema, namely low humidity, low ambient temperature, detergents and friction.

Generalized sweating tends to be increased because of the increased sensitivity to acetylcholine. It has been suggested – but not confirmed – that sweat retention plays a role in the itch. Patients with atopic eczema complain of excessive itching when hot (? and sweaty) in bed. Generally the hot red skin of atopic eczema feels dry unless the eczema is weeping or infected.

Thus the individual with atopic eczema cannot maintain a soft and pliable skin, exhibits cutaneous dryness, and readily chaps and fissures, especially in low relative humidity. Rubbing or scratching readily damages such skin, triggering the pruritic cycle.

PSYCHOLOGICAL FACTORS

While general practitioners are accustomed to consider the social and psychological factors, as well as the physical, in any illness, dermatologists are only too aware how easy it is to suggest psychological explanations for chronic skin diseases.

The evidence for an atopic personality is conflicting. Much of the difficulty lies in the fact that chronic pruritus and irritation can cause loss of sleep, irritability and restlessness, and the effectiveness of scratching in attracting attention is rapidly learnt. Maternal rejection by a distraught mother adds to the psychological disturbance and misery.

However, atopic eczema does appear to have a distinct tendency to flare in response to psychological stress. Patients subjected to experimental stress interviews showed erythema and then pruritus in skin areas subject to eczema.

SUMMARY OF ATOPIC ECZEMA

In response to allergic, physical and neural stimuli there is a release of histamine and other mast cell/basophil-associated mediators which is probably responsible for the acute phase of atopic eczema, causing erythema, severe pruritus and oedema.

The chronic phase is characterized by lichenification and marked xerosis. Many of the features of atopic eczema including excoriation and lichenification result from scratching and rubbing associated with pruritus.

Subsequent accumulation in the dermis of macrophages and T helper cells, with deficiency of T suppressor cells and excessive synthesis of IgE by B lymphocytes, imply disordered regulation of cell function in atopic eczema.

The cyclic nucleotide metabolic pathway, a major regulating system controlling mast cells and leukocytes is defective in atopic eczema. Basophils and mast cells from patients with atopic eczema release inappropriately high amounts of histamine in experimental conditions. Many of the dysfunctional immune and inflammatory abnormalities in atopic eczema may be the result of inadequate cyclic AMP inhibitory control of bone marrow-derived cells infiltrating into the dermis. Thus the fundamental defect in atopic eczema appears to be an impaired control of cell function of genetic origins. It is uncertain which of the various mechanisms discussed is primary, and which are secondary, since they all appear to react with each other.

REFERENCES

1. Russell Jones, R. (1982). P.E.E.P.O. papular eruption with elimination of papillary oedema. *Br. J. Dermatol.*, **106**, 393
2. Cunliffe, W. J. and Savin, J. A. (1986). In: Rook, A., Wilkinson, D. S., Ebling, F. J. G., Champion, R. H. and Burton, J. L. (eds), *Textbook of Dermatology*, 4th edn, p. 2247. (Oxford: Blackwell Scientific Publications)
3. Burton, J. L. and Pye, R. J. (1983). Seborrhoea is not a feature of seborrhoeic dermatitis. *Br. Med. J.*, **286**, 1169
4. Schuster, S. (1984). The aetiology of dandruff and the mode of action of therapeutic agents. *Br. J. Dermatol.*, **111**, 235
5. Ford, G. P. et al. (1984). The response of seborrhoeic dermatitis to ketoconazole. *Br. J. Dermatol.*, **111**, 603
6. Eisenstadt, B. A. and Wormser, E. P. (1984). Seborrhoeic dermatitis and butterfly rash in AIDS. *N. Engl. J. Med.*, **311**, 189
7. Vickers, C. F. H. (1980). The natural history of atopic eczema. *Acta Dermato-Venereol.*, Suppl. **92**, 113
8. Podmore, P. et al. (1986). Seborrhoeic eczema – a disease entity or a clinical variant of atopic eczema? *Br. J. Dermatol.*, **115**, 341
9. Browse, N. L. and Burnand, K. G. (1982). The cause of venous ulceration. *Lancet*, **2**, 243
10. Cronin, E. et al. (1980). In: Brown, S. S. and Sunderman, J. R. (eds), *Nickel Toxicology*, p. 149. (New York: Academic Press)
11. Jones, S. K. et al. (1987). Juvenile plantar dermatosis – an 8-year follow-up of 102 patients. *Clin. Exp. Dermatol.*, **12**, 5
12. Soter, N. A. and Mihm, M. C. Jr (1980). Morphology of atopic eczema. *Acta Dermato-Venereol.* Suppl. **92**, 11

13. Rajka, G. (1983). Atopic dermatitis. In: Rook, A. J. and Maibach, H. I. (eds), *Recent Advances in Dermatology*, No. 6, p. 110. (Edinburgh: Churchill Livingstone)

14. Schuster, D. L. et al. (1976) Selective deficiency of a T cell sub-population in active atopic dermatitis. *J. Immunol.*, **177**, 2171

15. Cooper, K. D. et al. (1980) Heterologous desensitisation of leucocytes – a possible mechanism of beta adrenergic blockade in atopic dermatitis. *Clin. Res.*, **28**, 566

16. Buckley, R. H. and Becher, W. G. (1978). Abnormalities in the regulation of human IgE synthesis. *Immunol. Rev.*, **41**, 288

17. Taylor, B., Norman, A. P., Orgel, H., Stokes, C. R., Turner, M. W. and Soothill, J. F. (1973). Transient IgA deficiency and pathogenesis of infantile atopy. *Lancet*, **2**, 111

18. Sillevis Smitt Bos J. et al. (1986). In situ immunophenotyping of antigen presenting cells and T cell subsets in atopic dermatitis. *Clin. Exp. Dermatol.*, **11**, 159–168

19. Safko, M. J., Chan, S. C., Cooper, K. D. and Hanifin, J. M. (1981). Heterologous desensitisations of leucocytes: a possible mechanism of beta-adrenergic blockade in atopic dermatitis. *J. Allergy Clin. Immunol.*, **68**, 218

20. Szentivanyi, A. (1968). The beta-adrenergic theory of the atopic abnormality in bronchial asthma. *J. Allergy*, **42**, 203

21. Dahl, M. V. (1983). *Staphylococcus aureus* and atopic dermatitis. *Arch. Dermatol.*, **119**, 840

22. Radermaher, M. and Maldague, M. P. (1981). Depression of neutrophil chemotaxis in atopic individual: an H_2 histamine response. *Int. Arch. Allergy*, **65**, 144

23. Welbourne, E., Champion, R. H. and Paris, W. E. (1981). Hypersensitivity to bacteria in eczema. *Br. J. Dermatol.*, **94**, 619

24. Lever, L. R., Leigh, D. A. and Wilkinson, J. (1985). A double blind study to assess the effectiveness of Mupirocin in the treatment of infected eczema. *Br. J. Dermatol.*, **113**, Suppl. 29, p. 35

25. Ohman, S., Juhlin, L. and Johansson, S. G. O. (1972). Immunoglobulins in atopic dermatitis. In *Allergology*. Proceedings of 8th European Congress of Allergy, p. 119. (Amsterdam: Excerpta Medica)

26. Mitchell, E. B., Crow, J., Williams, G. and Platts-Mills, T. A. E. (1986). Increase in skin mast cells following chronic house dust mite exposure. *Br. J. Dermatol.*, **114**, 65

27. Sampson, H. A. and Albergo, R. (1983). Comparison of results of skin, RAST and double blind placebo controlled challenge (DBFC) food tests in children with atopic dermatitis. (Presented at Annual Meeting of the American Academy of Allergology and Immunology, March 1983)

28. Taylor, B., Wadsworth, J., Wadsworth, M. and Peckham, C. (1984). Changes in the reported prevalence of childhood eczema since the 1939–'45 war. *Lancet*, **2**, 1255

29. Halpern, S. R., Sellars, W. A., Johnson, R. B., Anderson, D. W., Saperstein, S. and Reisch, J. S. (1973) Development of childhood allergy in infants fed breast, soya or cow's milk. *J. Allergy Clin. Immunol.*, **51**, 139

30. Atherton, D. J., Sewell, M., Soothill, J. F., Wells, R. S. and Chilvers, C. E. D. (1978). A double blind controlled cross-over trial of an antigen-avoidance diet in atopic eczema. *Lancet*, **1**, 401

31. Matthew, D. J., Taylor, B., Norman, A. P., Turner, M. W. and Soothill, J. F. (1977). Prevention of eczema. *Lancet*, **1**, 321

32. Sampson, H. A. (1983). Role of immediate food hypersensitivity in the pathogenesis of atopic dermatitis. *J. Allergy Clin. Immunol.*, **71**, 473

33. Jackson, P. G., Lessof, M. H., Baker, R. W. R. et al. (1981). Intestinal permeability in patients with eczema and food allergy. *Lancet*, **1**, 1285

34. Pike, M. and Atherton, D. (1987). In: Brostoff, J. and Challacombe, S. (eds), *Food Allergy and Intolerance*, p. 585. (London: Baillière Tindall)

Index

acetylcholine, effect in atopic eczema 180
acne, sebum secretion 169
acne rosacea 109
acrodermatitis continua 8, 16
adenosine monophosphate, cyclic (cAMP)
  atopic eczema 183–4
  cascade defects, in psoriasis 80–1
age of onset
  psoriasis 12
  psoriatic arthropathy 34
allergy
  atopic eczema 181, 187–8
  environmental causes 141
  sensitization 168–9
  to preservative in corticosteroid preparations 126
  see also contact eczema, allergic
alopecia areata, differential diagnosis 30
amcinolone acetonide 128
amyloidosis, with psoriatic arthropathy 36
anaemia, with psoriasis 24
ankylosing spondylitis 4, 32
  with psoriatic arthropathy 34, 35
anti-basal cell nuclear antibodies, in psoriasis 90
antibiotics, systemic 134–5

antihistamines, eczema treatment 140, 144
antimalarials, contraindicated for psoriatic arthropathy 36
antimicrobials, combined with corticosteroids 133–4
antiviral agents, systemic 135
arachidonic acid (AA), link with nucleotide pathways 83–5
arsenic ingestion, PUVA therapy contraindicated 49
arthropathy see psoriatic arthropathy
asteatotic eczema 106, 118
  aetiology 172–3
  management 154
asthma, with eczema 116
atopic eczema 106, 109
  aetiology 177–90
  allergy 187–8
  antihistamines 144
  bacterial infections 186–7
  cell-mediated immunity 185–6
  clinical features 114–16
  clothing 143
  desensitization 184–6
  diet 145–7
  effect of breast-feeding 188–9
  employment choices 143
  food exclusion and challenge 189–90
  hospital admission 145

atopic eczema – *cont.*
  lack of IgA 182
  lichenification 115
  management 142–50
  non-food allergens 147
  pharmacological effects 180
  physiological aspects 179
  prescribing 144–5
  psychological factors 148, 191
  self-limiting 143
  serum IgE levels 181–2
  skin abnormalities 190–1
  stress 191
  summary 191–2
  T suppressor cells 182
azathioprine
  psoriasis therapy 56–7
  psoriatic arthropathy 36

bacterial infections
  atopic eczema 186–7
  seborrhoeic eczema 170–1
  spread by corticosteroids 131
barrier creams 140
basal cell carcinoma, differential
  diagnosis 27
beta-blockers
  atopic eczema 184
  precipitating psoriasis 19, 82
betamethasone valerate 128
blepharitis 107–8, 152
bones, hyperostotic effects of etretinate
  53
Bowen's disease, differential diagnosis
  26
breast-feeding, effect on atopic eczema
  188–9

calcium, role in psoriasis 86
calmodulin, raised levels in psoriasis 86
Candida albicans infection 133
  differential diagnosis 28
capillaries
  in eczema 162
  in psoriasis 78–80
cardiac failure
  with exfoliative dermatitis 114
  with psoriasis 24
cellulitis, hypostatic eczema 112
chloroquine, precipitating psoriasis 19
clobetasol butyrate 127
clobetasol proprionate 128
contact eczema 76, 106

allergic 119–22
  aetiology 167–9
  clinical features 120–1
  corticosteroid side-effect 131
  management 156–7
  patch testing 121
irritant 118–19
  aetiology 165–7
  management 157–8
  secondary sites 112–13
corticosteroids
  contraindicated for psoriatic
    arthropathy 36
  precipitating psoriasis 19
  psoriasis therapy 45–7
  side-effects 46–7
  systemic 129–30, 134
  tachyphylaxis 46
  topical 123–34
    atopic eczema 144
    classification 126–8
    combination therapies 132–4
    composition 124–8
    guidelines for use 132
    mode of action 128
    preparations and potency 44
    prescribing 129–30
    reducing strength 132
    side-effects 124, 130–1
    types of preparation 124–5
counselling, psoriasis patients 39
cryotherapy, psoriasis 58
cyclosporin
  atopic eczema 183
  psoriasis therapy 57–8, 86
  psoriatic arthropathy 36
  side-effects 57–8

dandruff 107
Dead Sea bathing, psoriasis therapy 51
dermal cells
  eczema 162
  psoriasis 68
    pathogenesis 77–80
dermatitis, distinguished from eczema
  105
desoxymethasone 127, 128
dialysis, psoriasis therapy 58
diet
  atopic eczema 145–7
    allergens 188
    food exclusion and challenge 189–
      90

eczema management 141
and psoriasis 40
diflucortolone valerate 128
discoid eczema *see* nummular eczema
discoid lupus erythematosus 109
dithranol
  contraindications 43
  psoriasis therapy 43–5
  short-contact regimes 44–5
drugs
  eruptions
    differential diagnosis 28
    with exfoliative dermatitis 114
  hypersensitivity in atopic eczema
    116
  precipitating psoriasis 19, 74
  psoriasis therapy 51–8

eczema
  antibiotics and antivirals 134–5
  classification 105–6, 164–5
  clinical features, range 105
  course of disease 164
  craquelé *see* asteatotic eczema
  definition 161
  emollients 135–7
  environmental control 140–1
  histological changes 161–2
  hospital admission 141
  lichenification 110
  lotions, wet dressings and soaks 137
  paints 138
  paste bandages 139–40
  patterns of spread 163
  principles of management 142
  scarring 163
  secondary dissemination 112–13
  topical corticosteroids 123–34
  see also asteatotic eczema; atopic
    eczema; contact eczema;
    hypostatic eczema; juvenile
    plantar dermatosis; nummular
    eczema; perioral eczema;
    photosensitive eczema; pityriasis
    alba; pompholyx; seborrhoeic
    eczema
emollients 135–7, 140
epidemiology
  psoriasis 1–2
  psoriatic arthropathy 32–3
epidermal cells
  in eczema 162
  effect of hormone-like molecules 81

psoriasis 66, 67, 68
  hyperproliferation 69, 78, 91
  pathogenesis 76–7
  proliferation rate 74–6, 77
  T lymphocytes 70
epidermal proliferation factor (EPF)
  91
epidermal thymocyte-activating factor
  (ETAF) 91
erythrasma, differential diagnosis 28
erythroderma *see* exfoliative dermatitis
erythrodermic psoriasis 4
  clinical pattern 6–7
  differential diagnosis 29
  effect of corticosteroids 19
  hair loss 25
  hypothermia 23
  jaundice 23
  prognosis 15–16
  shivering 13
  therapy 15, 16
    etretinate 51, 52
erythroplasia of Queyrat, differential
  diagnosis 29
etretin 54
etretinate
  added to PUVA regime 50
  combined with PUVA or UVB 52
  psoriasis therapy 51–4
  side-effects 52–3
  teratogenicity 53
exfoliative dermatitis 106, 113–14
  management 159
eyes
  involvement in psoriatic arthropathy
    35
  psoriatic lesions 10

family studies, psoriasis 2–3
feet
  forefoot eczema 149
  juvenile plantar eczema 116–17
  see also pompholyx
fever, pustular psoriasis 13
fissures
  psoriasis 12
  seborrhoeic eczema 107, 108
flexural lesions
  atopic eczema 115
  seborrhoeic eczema 108
flexural psoriasis *see* intertriginous
  psoriasis
fluocinolone acetate 127, 128

folate deficiency, with psoriasis   24
folliculitis
    with seborrhoeic eczema   108
    with tar therapy   42
fungal infections
    intertriginous psoriasis   23
    seborrhoeic eczema   170–1

genetic factors
    atopic eczema   114, 178–9
    psoriasis   2–4
        capillaries   78–80
        fibroblasts   78
        skin defects   74–6
    psoriatic arthropathy   33
    pustular psoriasis   7
glaucoma, corticosteroids side-effect
    131
Goeckermann regime   41, 79–80
gold salts, psoriatic arthropathy   36
gravitation eczema see hypostatic
    eczema
guanosine monophosphate, cyclic
    (cGMP)
    atopic eczema   183–4
    in psoriatic epidermis   82
guttate psoriasis   7, 72–3
    clinical pattern   6
    differential diagnosis   27–8
    prognosis   15
    T cells   71

hair loss
    erythrodermic psoriasis   25
    etretinate side-effects   52
    exfoliative dermatitis   113
halcinonide   128
hands
    contact eczema   119, 120
    eczema see pomphylox
    nummular eczema   154
hay fever, with eczema   116
herpes simplex
    and atopic eczema   116
    with eczema, management   135
    spread by corticosteroids   131
histamine
    desensitization   185
    effect in atopic eczema   180
HLA studies, psoriasis   3–4
Hodgkin's disease, with exfoliative
    dermatitis   114
hormonal factors, precipitating

psoriasis   18, 74
hospital admission
    atopic eczema   145
    eczema   141
hydrocortisone   126, 127
5-hydroxy urea, psoriasis therapy   56
hyperkeratosis, subungual   11, 30–1
hyperthermia, with psoriasis   24
hypoalbuminaemia, with psoriasis   25
hypoparathyroidism, exacerbating
    psoriasis   18
hypostatic eczema   106
    aetiology   173–4
    clinical features   111–12
    management   152–3
    secondary sites   112
hypothermia
    with exfoliative dermatitis   114
    with psoriasis   23

ichthyosis   114
id reaction   110
    aetiology   175–6
immunology
    atopic eczema   180–6
    contact allergic eczema   119–20
    hormonal effects   18
    psoriasis   3–4
        cellular components   90–6
        non-cellular components   87–90
        pathogenesis   86–96
    psoriatic arthropathy   33
    seborrhoeic eczema   171
indomethacin, precipitating psoriasis
    19
infections
    precipitating psoriasis   17–18, 71
    secondary to psoriasis   23
inflammatory bowel disease, with
    psoriatic arthropathy   35
interferon
    effect on DNA synthesis, psoriatic
        skin   76–7
    effect on keratinocytes   76
intertriginous lesions, seborrhoeic
    eczema   108
intertriginous psoriasis   9
    differential diagnosis   28
    fungal infections   23
    pain   12
iron deficiency, with psoriasis   24
itching
    antihistamines   140

eczema 162
    atopic 177–8
    exfoliative dermatitis 113
    psoriasis 12

jaundice, with erythrodermic
    psoriasis 23
juvenile eczemas
    atopic 115
    perioral 117
    plantar 116–17, 176
    seborrhoeic 109
juvenile plantar dermatosis 106, 116–
    17

Kaposi's varicelliform eruption 116,
    185
keratinization, abnormalities in
    psoriasis 69
keratinocytes 91
keratolytics
    combined with corticosteroids 134
    eczema treatment 138
keratosis pilaris 114
kidneys, cyclosporin toxicity 57
Koebner reaction 20, 31, 87, 89, 91

Langerhans cells 71, 90, 167, 168
laser surgery, psoriasis 58
lichen planus 76
    differential diagnosis 26, 29, 30
lichen simplex 111, 128
    differential diagnosis 25
    management 156
lichen striatus 148
lichenification
    atopic eczema 115
    eczema 110, 162
lithium, exacerbating psoriasis 19, 81–
    2, 95
liver
    disorders, with psoriasis 23
    etretinate side-effects 53
    methotrexate toxicity 54
lymph nodes, exfoliative dermatitis
    113
lymphoma, with exfoliative dermatitis
    114

malignancy, and methotrexate
    therapy 55
marrow toxicity
    azathioprine 57

5-hydroxy urea 56
melanoma, malignant, PUVA therapy
    contraindicated 49
menopause, precipitating psoriasis 18
mepacrine, precipitating psoriasis 19
methotrexate
    combined with etretinate 52
    psoriasis therapy 54–6, 86
    psoriatic arthropathy 36
    side-effects 55–6
mobility, loss in psoriasis 13
moisturizers 136–7
monoclonal antibodies, study of T cell
    antigens 70
monocytes, abnormal function in
    psoriasis 94–5
mouth
    perioral eczema 117
    psoriatic lesions 10
Munro abscesses 66, 67, 89
mycosis fungoides
    differential diagnosis 26–7
    with exfoliative dermatitis 114

nails
    exfoliative dermatitis 113
    in psoriasis 10–11
        differential diagnosis 30
        link with arthropathy 35
        pitting 10
        prognosis 16
    'napkin dermatitis' 109, 172
    'napkin psoriasis' 172
neomycin, and secondary eczema 113
neutrophils, in psoriasis
    effect of stratum corneum
        antibodies 89
    peripheral blood counts 95
    role in pathogenesis 95–6
non-steroidal anti-inflammatories
    precipitating psoriasis 19
    psoriatic arthropathy 36
nucleotides, cyclic
    link with arachidonic acid pathway
        85
    role in skin defects in psoriasis 80–2
nummular eczema 106, 115
    aetiology 176
    clinical features 111
    differential diagnosis 26
    management 153–4

oedema, with psoriasis 24

oncholysis 11, 30
ornithine decarboxylase (ODC), role in
    psoriasis 82
otitis externa, with seborrhoeic
    eczema 108

pain, intertriginous psoriasis 12
paints, eczema treatment 138
palmo-plantar psoriasis, etretinate
    therapy 52
palmo-plantar pustulosis 7
palms
    eczema see pompholyx
    psoriasis 9, 12
        differential diagnosis 29
parakeratosis, in psoriasis 66, 69
paste bandages, eczema 139–40
patch testing
    contact allergic eczema 121
    photosensitive eczema 122
pemphigus 109
penis, psoriatic lesions 10, 29
perioral eczema 117
photosensitive dermatitis 106
photosensitive eczema 122
    management 158–9
phototherapy, psoriasis 47–51
pityriasis alba 106, 117, 148–9
pityriasis lichenoides chronica,
    differential diagnosis 28
pityriasis rosea, differential diagnosis
    27
pityriasis rubea pilaris, differential
    diagnosis 27
Pityrosporon ovale infection 170–1
plaque psoriasis 7
    clinical pattern 5
    differential diagnosis 25–7
    precipitated by beta-blockers 82
    prognosis 14–15
    progression to erythrodermic 6
plasma abnormalities, in psoriasis 89
plasminogen activator, involved and
    uninvolved skin, in psoriasis 73
polyamines, role in psoriasis 82–3
pompholyx 106
    aetiology 174–5
    clinical features 109–10
    management 155
potassium permanganate soaks 137
pregnancy
    effect of psoriasis 18
    PUVA therapy contraindicated 49

teratogenicity of etretinate 53
teratogenicity of methotrexate 55
prognoses
    psoriasis 14–17
        active and stable states compared
            21
    psoriatic arthropathy 36
proteinases, role in psoriasis 85–6
psoriasis
    acrodermatitis continua 8
        prognosis 16
    active state 21–2
    aetiology 65, 71–2
    age of onset 12
    characteristic features 66
    complications 22–5
    defects of cell-mediated immunity
        92
    differential diagnosis 25–31, 108
    epidemiology 1–2
    excoriation of scale 4–5
    with exfoliative dermatitis 114
    genetic factors 2–4
    histology of plaques 66–8
    historical background 1
    inactive state 21
    management 39
    morphology of lesions 4–5
    mucosal lesions 10
    nail lesions 10–11
    natural history and prognosis 14–17
    nature of cellular infiltrate 69–71
    pathogenesis 72
    persistence of lesions 86, 91
    precipitating factors 17–20
    psychosocial factors 13–14
    response to mitogens 92–4
    symptoms 12–13
    T cell-mediated disease 91
    see also erythrodermic psoriasis;
        guttate psoriasis; pustular psoriasis
psoriatic arthropathy 31–2
    clinical features 33–4
    cyclosporin therapy 57
    definition 32
    epidemiology 32–3
    extra-articular features 35
    genetic factors 33
    link with nail involvement 35
    link with pustular psoriasis 35
    prognosis 36
    relationship with psoriatic lesions 35
    treatment 36

psychological factors
  atopic eczema 116, 148, 191
  family support 142–3
  in pompholyx 110
  psoriasis 13–14
    counselling 39
puberty, precipitating psoriasis 18
pustular psoriasis
  clinical pattern 7–8
  differential diagnosis 30
  effect of corticosteroids 19
  etretinate therapy 51, 52
  exacerbated by beta-blockers 82
  fever 13
  prognosis 16
  psoriasis 35
  secondary infections 23
putrescine, role in psoriasis 82
PUVA (psoralens + ultraviolet A)
  atopic eczema 150
  combined with corticosteroids 46
  combined with etretinate 52
  eczema 142
  psoriasis therapy 47–50, 86
    effect on capillaries 79–80
  psoriatic arthropathy 36
  therapy side-effects 49–50

Reiter's disease, link with psoriasis 4
remissions, length of 15, 21
renal disorders, with psoriasis 25
reverse Koebner reaction 87
ringworm infection
  differential diagnosis 28, 31
  pompholyx diagnosis 110
rupioid lesions 5, 9

sacroiliitis, associated with psoriasis 34
sarcoidosis 109
scalp
  corticosteroid preparations 125
  dandruff 107
  eczema 107
  psoriasis 8
    differential diagnosis 30
    scaling 13
  shampoos 138, 151
  tar preparations 42
scratch marks 105–6
scratching, white dermographism 115,
  179–80
seborrhoea 169
seborrhoeic eczema 106

adult 107–9
  management 151–2
aetiology 169–71, 171–2
differential diagnosis 25, 28, 29, 30,
  108–9
immunology 171
infantile 109
  management 150–1
serum abnormalities, in psoriasis 87–9
shampoos 138, 151
shivering, erythrodermic psoriasis 13
skin
  abnormalities, atopic eczema 190–1
  ageing effect of PUVA therapy 49
  barrier to irritant contact eczema
    165–6
  consequences of damage 166–7
  defects in psoriasis
    genetic factors 74–80
    molecular nature 80–6
  factors weakening barrier role 166
  psoriasis
    scaling 13
    uninvolved 31, 72
  retinoid dermatitis 52
  trauma, precipitating psoriasis 20,
    72
  white dermatographism 115, 179–80
soaks 137
soap substitutes 136
social factors, psoriasis 13–14
soles, psoriasis 9, 12
  differential diagnosis 29
spermidine, role in psoriasis 82
spinal arthritis, link with psoriasis 34
Staphylococcus aureus infections 133,
  135
stratum corneum 166
  antibodies, in psoriasis 89–90
streptococcal infections, precipitating
  psoriasis 17, 91–2
stress
  atopic eczema 191
  exacerbating seborrhoeic eczema
    171
  precipitating psoriasis 18–19, 39, 72
subcorneal pustular dermatosis,
  differential diagnosis 30
surgery
  psoriasis therapy 58
  psoriatic arthropathy 36
syphilis, secondary, differential
  diagnosis 27

T cells
  atopic eczema   182, 183
  in psoriasis   69–71, 90–4
    in uninvolved skin   72
tar
  combined with corticosteroids   134
  eczema treatment   139
  psoriasis therapy   40–2
therapy
  erythrodermic psoriasis   15, 16
  immunosuppressive activity   86
  length of subsequent remissions   15, 21
  psoriasis
    dialysis   58
    drugs   51–8
    phototherapy   47–51
    surgery   58
    topical   40–7
  risks involved   16–17
trauma, precipitating psoriasis   20
triamcinolone acetonide   129
triamcinolone diacetate   130
triamcinolone hexacetonide,
  intralesional injection   46

triglyceride levels, etretinate side-
  effects   52–3
twin studies, psoriasis   3

ulcers, leg, hypostatic eczema   112
ultraviolet B
  combined with corticosteroids   46
  combined with etretinate   52
  psoriasis therapy   51
ultraviolet light
  psoriasis therapy   41, 42, 51
  see also PUVA; ultraviolet B

vaccinia virus, and atopic eczema   116
varicose eczema see hypostatic eczema
varicose veins, hypostatic eczema   111
vasodilatation, precipitating
  psoriasis   77
virus-like particles, in psoriatic lesions
  91
vitamin A
  results in psoriasis   51
  see also etretinate

wet dressings   137